THE NEW
5 DAYS TO A
FLATTER
STOMACH

Also by Monica Grenfell

Fabulous in a Fortnight

Monica's Fabulous Body Plan: Fantastic Legs & Thighs

Monica's Fabulous Body Plan: Best Bust, Arms and Back

Monica's Fabulous Body Plan: Marvellous Midriff

Monica's Fabulous Body Plan: Beautiful Bottom

Beat Your Body Chaos

Cellulite Buster: the 30-Day Diet

The New Get Back Into Your Jeans Diet

THE NEW
5 DAYS TO A
FLATTER
STOMACH

Beat the Bulge and Banish Bloating

MONICA GRENFELL

PAN BOOKS

Advice to the reader

Before following any medical or
dietary advice contained in this
book, it is recommended that
you consult your doctor if you
suffer from any health problems
or special conditions or are in
any doubt as to its suitability.

First published 1997 as *5 Days to a Flatter Stomach* by Boxtree.

This edition published 2004 by Pan Books
an imprint of Pan Macmillan Ltd
Pan Macmillan, 20 New Wharf Road, London N1 9RR
Basingstoke and Oxford
Associated companies throughout the world
www.panmacmillan.com

ISBN 0 330 43276 1

9 8 7 6 5 4 3 2 1

A CIP catalogue record for this book is available from
the British Library.

Printed and bound in Great Britain by The Bath Press

contents

To my sister Shelagh

Monica's Mailbag

Let me know how you are getting on,
tell me what problems you have and share
with me how successful you have been in
achieving a flatter stomach!

Email me via my website:
www.monicagrenfell.co.uk

or write to me at:

Monica's Mailbag,
PO Box 64,
Oxon OX12 9GA

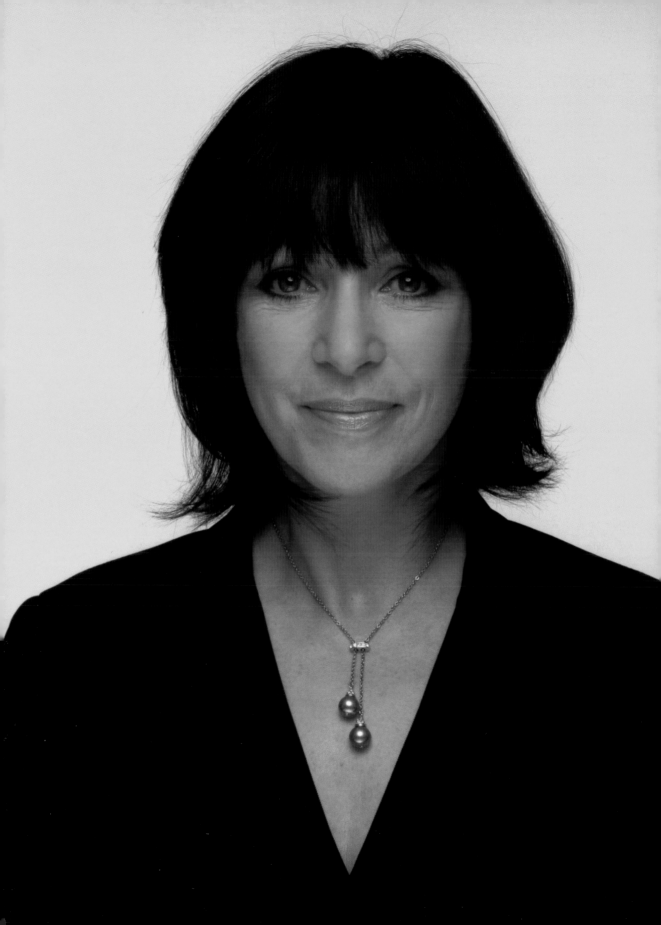

Foreword

Hello, I am Monica Grenfell and this is my **New 5 Days to a Flatter Stomach**.

How much do you really want a flatter stomach? Maybe you have been fighting the battle for years as you embark on yet another diet and shell out for gym memberships. Things go well for a while and you lose weight. But your stomach stays stubbornly bloated and uncomfortable, as if some bloat-beast decides to visit, just when you least expected him. How can this happen when you have done all the right things, like exercising and cutting calories?

If all this sounds uncomfortably familiar, you have come to the right place – because I had a serious relationship with the bloat-beast for years. The fact that I beat it is the reason for this book.

Every night for ten years, I squeezed myself into a skintight leotard and leggings and stood in front of 100 pairs of critical eyes as I taught exercise classes. When people are gazing at your stomach, thighs, arms and any other bits which might be flapping in the breeze, night after night, year after year, you learn a few tricks. I dreaded a bloated stomach. My day revolved around making sure it was flat by evening. And this was quite a task. I do not teach fitness these days, but as a qualified nutritionist with the most read magazine column in the country, I know from my massive mailbag that your stomach area is the most hated area of the body. You are probably in despair over the bloating, discomfort and sheer size, in comparison with the rest of your body. I am sure you work hard at it and, believe me, I understand how you feel. After two children (one caesarean) and a couple of stomach operations, not to mention the fact that I am not as young as I was, it is quite a feat to have a flat stomach. But I have, and it is entirely due to this programme, which I have developed over many years.

A great body is worth working at. Never believe the doom-mongers who say you can't hope to have a good figure after babies or a flat stomach after forty. You can. The Grenfell 5-Day programme is an amalgamation of all I have learned. I know you are going to be delighted with it and will want to follow the programme into the future.

Good luck, and never despair. You can do it!

Monica Grenfell

Introduction

Every woman wants a flat stomach.
Whether or not you champion
voluptuous curves, a womanly bottom
or a statuesque bosom, nobody wants
a big stomach. The success of the first
edition of my programme prompted this
new version, brought up to date but still
containing all the elements that made
it a hit first time around. A few tricks of
the trade, an amazing diet and a good
5-point programme to help you manage
that stomach for the rest of your life.

So what brings you here? Maybe you
have a food intolerance or have been
transformed by your pregnancies. Are
you bloated beyond what is tolerable?
Do you eat because you are happy, or
comfort-eat because you are sad? It is
a shame to be dissatisfied with your life.
You can spend a fortune on designer
labels and fill your bathroom with
expensive cosmetics, but these just
paper over the cracks. If only you felt
completely confident about your body,
you could pull on a pair of old jeans and
everyone would admire you. But if you
feel fat or bloated you can dress from
top to toe in Chanel and still feel
awful inside.

Diets *do* work

Diets don't work if you stop doing them. How could
they! To explain why you gain weight again after a diet,
look at this analogy: a footballer keeps suffering from
a knee injury; his playing style is analysed and he is
told that he is running and kicking the wrong way. He
goes for an operation and is out of the game for six
months. He comes back and plays the same way as
before, in the same shoes and on the same surfaces.
Guess what – the injury comes back.

If you do the *same* things in the *same* way, you will
get the same results. If your old ways made you pile
on the pounds, what can you expect if you go back to
doing what you were before?

But you have to be sensible. Men don't fall for your
fat ratio. Friends can't see your weight. Serving yourself with fat-free alternatives like a second-class
citizen while the rest of the family eats the real thing
isn't necessary, and on this diet you won't be doing it.
I don't want a diet to be so different and quirky from
normal life that you draw attention to yourself. For the
first time I have taken the stress out of slimming and
brought back reality. Reality means food people really
want to eat. Reality means not having to spend ten
minutes packing a holdall with equipment and changing into special gear just to go and exercise. Reality
means admitting that we don't want to just eat
mounds of protein.

5 DAYS – are you serious ?

Of course I am serious!

It takes just five days to settle that stomach and lose excess fluids. In only five days your muscles can be more toned and supple than they have felt for years. The diet is safe and probably healthier than you have eaten for a while. The programme takes you into the future and the work will have to be kept up, but the possibilities will delight you:

For example, you have probably been told to do the following:

- breakfast like a king, lunch like a prince and dine like a pauper
- eat plenty of fruit and vegetables
- eat nothing after 6 p.m.
- start the day with a good breakfast
- nibble on dried fruit for energy
- drink diet drinks instead of the sugary versions
- cut fat
- use low-sugar versions of desserts and sweets.

But on the 5-Day programme you will have the following:

- four small snacks during the day
- most food after 6 p.m.
- no fruit and few vegetables during the day
- no dried fruit, except a few prunes in the evening
- no fizzy or diet drinks
- normal-fat foods, like butter and cheese
- no artificial sweeteners.

Those are some big changes!

Yes, but you will love them. The biggest blocks to starting something new are fear, scepticism and idleness. Fear that doing something new will disrupt your routine, scepticism because you have tried so many things and they didn't work, and idleness – well, we are all idle about something. Suddenly a year has gone by and you realize you never made that telephone call, wrote that letter or started that diet. But what's the bottom line in all this? Having a flatter stomach. It's why you bought this book. You want it more than anything else, so don't let a few old habits get in the way.

The Grenfell Philosophy

Feeling happy and confident about your figure is your pathway to success. I truly believe this. People who struggle to be slim, even if they profess not to care, are rarely happy and confident inside. They will often try to buy their way to happiness, with designer labels, extravagant shoes and expensive beauty treatments.

Being is more important than *having*. My philosophy is that beauty is the entire effect, and all your clothes and make-up are nothing if you feel fat and unhealthy. Start with the underneath. Don't eat food that clogs your insides and don't pollute yourself with cigarettes and alcohol. What you are is more important than what you have, and if you are healthy, fit and glowing with confidence, you will attract people to you whether or not you are wearing designer clothes or drive a smart car.

And don't you want to give yourself an edge over others? It is not about looking like a celebrity or trying to copy your best friend. It is about presenting the best version of yourself. My simple 5-point programme will help you to achieve this. It will help you to remind yourself of your goals and revisit them constantly. This is not about me telling you what to do or what to think; it is about *you* telling you what to do and think. You set your own goals and you decide how you are going to achieve them. The Grenfell programme simply gives you the framework. And it really works!

I devised the Grenfell philosophy from mastering my own mind–body connection. It has enabled me to stay the same weight and shape for more than thirty years. I can truly say that I have never gained a pound or increased my vital statistics in all that time, and this certainly is not down to luck. Like you, I have to work at it. Like you, I need a proper diet. I have my bottom line, which I repeat frequently – that I want to be healthy and confident. The reassuring point for you, I hope, is that it has not made me self-obsessed or manic about my weight – far from it. Once you have your programme in place you will not be obsessed, because your body takes care of itself. You learn that beauty is the entire effect, nobody can see your weight and it is OK to have that chocolate. Chocolate's in the programme!

It all starts here

The programme starts with *The New 5 Days to a Flatter Stomach*. You are probably a diet veteran and already have your eagle eyes peeled for the get-out clause. You're probably used to the scenario where you lose those vanity pounds only to have them creep back on in the following days or weeks. Well, this is not a fad and it isn't a con. This is the 5-Day promise:

You will:

• banish bloating

• lose inches from waist and abdomen

• increase energy

• sleep better

• be more confident

• feel healthier.

And the plus-side is that so much of this plan re-introduces foods that die-hard dieters thought were off the menu for good. Butter and cheese. Rice pudding and potatoes. Seasoned slimmers will have already shrunk from the idea, convinced that their weight will soar overnight and the whole thing will end in tears. But give it five days and I promise you'll be amazed.

Tried and tested

I have been putting clients through this programme for years, but for the purposes of this book, I asked another 200 women who wanted to lose weight to try the plan.

None of the testers had any idea what the pro-gramme was aiming to achieve, only that I was trialling a diet-and-exercise plan for a book. They all kept diaries for me, as I was interested not only in changes in their weight and improvement, but also in whether the meals worked, whether their families enjoyed them and whether they could find the foods easily. It is no good suggesting a regime which puts people to endless trouble, or stipulating food that can't be taken to work.

The detailed responses of some of the team are contained in the next section (page 10). However, the diaries showed that:

• all the testers lost weight

• all the testers felt noticeably and pleasingly slimmer

• all the testers had managed to give up any laxatives and stomach medicines they had been taking for wind, and were thrilled at how calming the diet was

• all the testers said they could happily stick with the regime

• all the testers said they were pleased and relieved to be able to eat 'proper' food again – such as butter, eggs and cheese

• nobody disliked the diet in any way.

I believe I cannot go better than the evidence of those 200 volunteers who put themselves through my 5-Day programme and my grateful thanks go out to them all. Don't be sceptical. If such results can be achieved in only five days, think what you can achieve in a month!

Is This You? The Reasons People Don't Stick with a Diet

1 I don't see results quickly enough

Crash diets used to be a quick way of losing weight and cheering yourself up, but they gave you false hopes. If you lost six pounds (2.7kg) in your first week, a three-pound (1.4kg) loss the following week felt like failure. Only one and a half pounds (0.7kg) lost the next time and you were nearly suicidal. Never mind that this is perfectly standard weight loss – to you it felt like total standstill. Why be hungry, you reasoned, when nothing was happening? Focusing only on the downside, you forgot that six pounds off was good in itself. 'I ought to have lost a stone by now!' you moaned. Well, cheer up. The beauty of this diet is real inch loss. Seeing and feeling a real difference is a major psychological boost, which is why the 5-Day programme is so popular. This is not a crash diet, but the results are swift.

2 I used to be slim and be able to lose weight easily – now I'm older, the weight just won't go. What's happening? It's not fair!

Look, I want to be ten years younger too, but it isn't going to happen! We all did a lot of things differently when we were younger and, yes, now you have to run hard just to stay in the same place. But I promise that once you get into the 5-Day programme you'll be slim, vigorous and glad you made the effort.

Never mind what your age is, or that you've just had your fourth baby or that operation. Even if you are eighty, you can lose weight. If you take hormone tablets or have thyroid malfunction or you are Type 1 diabetic, you can still lose weight. Feeling that you are somehow a 'special' case is a cop-out. It's easy to blame circumstances for your not losing weight. If you start finding reasons why life used to be so much better, you'll never stop.

3 I reach a plateau and there doesn't seem to be any point

Yes, there is. Every scientific test I have ever seen has found that under strict conditions people lost weight at a continuous rate. There is no such thing as a plateau and everyone can lose the amount of weight they wish to lose – as long as they have excess body fat.

So take heart – you can lose those last ten pounds (4.5kg) with the Grenfell Maintenance programme.

4 I have to make one meal for myself and another for the rest of the family

My meals can be enjoyed by everyone. I don't use any low-calorie or low-fat alternatives, although some recipes are adapted to reduce thoughtless and liberal use of fattening ingredients. There is no need to treat yourself as a second-class citizen just because you want to lose weight. We all appreciate quality, and that means real butter, cheese and cream. As a guide, ask yourself what kind of dessert you would give to a guest. The lowest-calorie version or the richest? Many of the meals on this diet are standard favourites, which old and young alike can enjoy.

5 I feel hungry all the time

On this diet, you will be eating five or six times a day. The secret is to eat *small amounts of food regularly*. Ever woken at 3 a.m. feeling bright and wide awake, only to fall back to sleep and crawl out of bed in the morning feeling terrible? This is classic low blood sugar. My mid-evening supper gives you a restful sleep and you'll wake feeling refreshed.

6 I feel washed out and tired

Calorie-reduced or low-carbohydrate diets can make you very tired, as you are not putting any energy into your body. The 5-Day diet is completely different, because the staple daytime foods, while being light, are carbohydrates, and your daily intake of carbohydrate will be quite high. Your main meal, in particular, will be based on starchy carbohydrates, so you will feel energetic on the programme.

7 I feel bloated on all that fruit and fibre

Fruit is *meant* to fill you. It contains fibre and water and it flushes out your system wonderfully. If you have a constipation problem, eat fruit. However, there is a problem, because much fruit contains sorbitol, a natural sweetener that can cause bloating. If your stomach feels lovely and flat in the morning but bloated by early evening and you have been eating fruit, you've found the culprit. On this diet, you will simply shift all that wonderful fruit to the evening, out of harm's way.

How You Will Succeed

You are probably dying to know the secret by now. Well, hold on a little longer while I explain the simple methods to achieving that flatter stomach by the end of the week.

Limited Choice

If your kitchen usually looks like a harvest festival the minute you start a new diet, with your fridge over-flowing with fruits and vegetables, you are already on the way to failure. Stocking up on a huge variety of foods is a key to overeating, and scientific research has shown that when you are presented with a wide variety of choices, you will eat more.

The Grenfell programme presents you with a few key foods as part of a greatly simplified diet. Any time you are faced with those all-you-can-eat buffets, go for just two or three items rather than a bit of everything.

Going Low – Sodium, That Is

Don't get me wrong – your body needs sodium. It's a mineral that helps the body regulate blood pressure. It's also needed for muscle and nerve function. But you only need around 500–1,000mg a day and that is the amount in one smoked sausage!

And if you want to put a stop to that bothersome bloating, don't dread the bread –the problem is more likely to be sodium overload. You see, salt stimulates the taste buds, making you want an opposing taste. The more salt you have, the more likely you are to want sugar. The more sugar you eat, the more you will crave something sharp, bitter or salty. Simple food takes some getting used to, but it is surely better to have a basic diet, say, during the week, if you know it will help to stop cravings. Save your all-out curry night for a treat.

However, before you ban savouries, be aware that there is also a lot of salt in sweet foods like chocolate and cereals.

There is more sodium in a cup of Raisin Bran cereal (486mg) than in a cup of dry-roasted peanuts (9mg).

So go and check out your larder and read food labels: a low-sodium food contains no more than 140mg of sodium per serving.

These are all high in sodium:

- table salt

- seasonings that contain salt
  (celery salt, onion salt, etc.)

- tinned vegetables in brine

- pickles, including olives

- regular canned soups

- breads and rolls with salt toppings

- crisps, corn chips, pretzels, saltines, salty crackers,
  salted popcorn

- salty or smoked meats
  (bacon, corned beef, frankfurters, ham, luncheon
  meats, salt pork, sausage, canned or pickled
  meats)

- salty or smoked fish
  (anchovies, herring, sardines)

- processed cheese, cheese spreads, salty cheeses
  (Roquefort, Camembert, Gorgonzola, Parmesan)

- salted nuts

- peanut butter

- ketchup, chilli sauces, meat extracts, monosodium
  glutamate, mustard, soy sauce, Worcester sauce

- antacids containing sodium

- baking-soda toothpaste.

Don't worry if this appears to leave very little. You can still be creative with spices, herbs and even wine and spirits to give your meals flavour.

Nobody ever felt worse for exercising properly. The danger is setting yourself too high a goal and going at it like a bull at a gate. If you start on day one promising yourself an hour's aerobics and 500 sit-ups every day, you'll feel a failure when you can't keep it up.

My exercise plan combines a bit of the old, in crunches and standard sit-ups, with something new and exciting. The GrenFlex exercise band is simple and easy to use, but the results it gives are astounding. Flex bands are not new, but to date they have not really captured the nation's consciousness. That is about to change. The exercise section of this book includes a few fantastic flex exercises that absolutely anybody can do.

Do remember that your midsection forms a circle. When you exercise the abdominal muscles on their own, two-thirds of that circle sits idle. On the Grenfell programme, you will be toning your waist muscles and your back to provide a strong, balanced centre, lifting and toning your entire torso for pleasing posture and a tight tummy.

Posture stretches

However good your muscles are, however slim you have become, if you stand and sit badly your stomach will hang out. Every day of the programme includes posture stretches to maintain good body alignment, which alone can make you appear inches slimmer.

No Substitutes for the Best Foods

'I can't believe I'll be eating butter!' said one of my testers. 'My last diet banned cheese completely,' said another, adding that a lifetime without her favourite cheese-and-pickle sandwich wouldn't be worth living. I agree with her.

Nobody sticks with a menu plan stuffed with 'healthy alternatives'. The alternatives are often not healthy; in fact, they're often crammed so full of additives the list of ingredients takes up half the packaging. Yes, my diet insists on proper butter, half-fat crème fraiche, cheese and eggs, but it is a long way from being a high-protein diet. When the nation has been existing on a diet of crisps, hot dogs, bags of sweets, ice cream and pizza, washed down with lager or fizzy drinks, this diet is the healthiest food some people will have eaten for years!

Two-speed diet choice

My diet plan comes in two speeds:

1 **The Grenfell 5 Days to a Flatter Stomach programme** – this can be done for any five days you like, whenever you want a flatter stomach fast

2 **The Grenfell Lifetime Maintenance programme** – the full, 5-step programme to ensure you lose weight, achieve a better shape *and* keep your flatter stomach for good!

The 5-Day programme is very specific about what to eat and it guarantees fantastic results. The Maintenance programme offers slightly more choice and features my 5-point programme to remind you of your commitment. If you want to know how to keep up the good eating habits you've learned, this diet offers more meal choices and variety, and you'll continue to lose weight steadily as long as you have excess body fat.

Half the battle is your determination. Going for a few walks and eating smaller meals isn't hard, but if you hate going out and love your local takeaway it's going to take a shift in attitude. *Do* keep at it. No woman was ever sorry she lost a spare tyre. No woman ever looked back wistfully to her 'fat' days when she felt bloated and self-conscious.

Good luck!

Success Stories

How the Testers Got On

My whole weight-loss concept is so different from most diets, I wanted to put a team of testers through it. Not just to prove it worked, but to see if it was practical. After all, it's no good going embarking on a punishing regime that makes the whole family suffer, and nobody wants a sandwich lunch that is soggy by the time you get to work. I put the word out in my magazine column and literally thousands of women came forward to test the plan.

I chose a cross-section of people. A couple of women wanted to lose at least two stone (12.7kg), several testers reported few problems with their weight, but despair with their stomachs after having babies, and the majority simply wanted to lose about seven to ten pounds (3.2–4.5kg) and tone up their muscles. They all kept diaries for me, and I'm delighted to report that their results exceeded my wildest expectations. Here is a selection of their verdicts:

Irene Norton, forty-two, a medical secretary, is married with four teenage children

'I had to let you know straight away how completely thrilled I was with the Grenfell programme. I needed to lose more than a stone (6.4kg), but I find conventional diets too long-winded and not really practical for long-term use.

'At first I thought "Five days! I'll believe it when I see it!" but because my problem has always been psychological – I suppose I want instant success or I get disheartened – this was the perfect plan for me because I *felt* so much slimmer by the end of just three days, and that spurred me on.

'I had to give up the diet for a long weekend because we went away for a wedding, and I realized how awful I'd always felt before. It's the bloating, I think, and when your stomach's wrong you feel wrong all over. I've now gone back to it and I'm following the Grenfell Maintenance programme, which is incredibly do-able. I have lost twelve pounds (5.4kg) in five weeks, gone down a dress size and, most important, lost a lot of inches.

'To tell the truth, I couldn't care less about what the scales say, I'm more interested in how my clothes look, and my eldest daughter said yesterday that I looked ten years younger now I'm back to cinching in my waist with a nice belt.

'I'm really proud of my figure now, the diet's wonderful and I'll keep on the maintenance plan for good. It's nice to have someone spell it all out for you.'

Maria Telling, eighteen, is single and a sociology student at Manchester University

'The exercises worked best for me. I'm very untoned as I'm lazy about exercise, and my stomach had got quite flabby. Knowing there was only five minutes of exercising meant that I wasn't reluctant to do it, and although it wasn't easy, it worked! I was particularly thrilled with the flex bands. I haven't used anything like them before and I'm quite addicted now! They have toned up my lower stomach quite beautifully in just eight weeks.

'I didn't believe that you could do so much without going to an aerobics class for an hour a time, but I can honestly say that after five days I had an entirely different shape. I hold myself better too and I think that's made a huge difference.

'As far as the food was concerned, it was perfect. I'm sharing a flat that has an ancient oven and only two electric rings, so anything complicated was obviously out. I've also got no money! I spent far less on this diet than I usually do eating at the subsidized refectory at college, and my favourite meal was the spaghetti bolognese, because we could all share it, and it cost about five pounds for four of us, which was brilliant.'

Siobhan Everitt, thirty, is married with three children under five

'The Grenfell 5-Day programme is great. I wanted to lose about half a stone (3.2kg) and have tried a lot of diets, but this is the first one I'd stuck with. I suffer from irritable bowel syndrome, which blows me out, but with this diet I was so much better, with less wind and grumbling feelings. I think it was because it wasn't just fruit, fruit, fruit, which always makes me feel quite empty.

'I have to work hard at keeping slim, because with three children there's always the wrong food around and you're always making something. I'll have a Mars Bar in the afternoon because I'm starving, then I'll think, "Oh, I can't have any tea because I ate that chocolate", so I'm hungry again in the evening and eat a load of biscuits, so really it's a lot of rubbish I'm eating. And so it goes on.

'With the Grenfell programme, the food is so enjoyable. I felt I learned a lot, too. It was nice to eat more in the evening after so many years of being told you can't eat after 6 p.m. The most valuable part about it was the philosophy of the Maintenance programme. Monica asked many questions that hit the nail right on the head. Having a "bottom line" and a 5-point programme to follow meant I could remind myself continually of what this was all about and bring myself back in line. I liked that.

'I loved the avocado pear. I have never eaten one before and I thought, "I'm not sure about this, but it's on the diet", so I tried it with the prawns. It was wonderful!

'I'm carrying on with the programme from now on. I lost four pounds (1.8kg) and my stomach seems so much slimmer. I won't eat the old way ever again.'

Gillian Jaworsky, thirty-five, is an actress, married without children

'I admit to being obsessed with my body, and I notice every millimetre on it. My husband and I entertain, so I was a bit worried I'd either be stuck with ghastly hotpots or have to give up the diet altogether when we entertained. How wrong I was! I could eat smoked salmon and crème fraiche, and the cheese soufflé was out of this world!

'I'm an intermittent, picky eater. I also binge, then starve for days because I feel wretched. I suppose it is because I am in the theatre and my job means looking good and it's quite stressful. I tend to go for three days being good, then I eat a square of chocolate and think I might as well eat the lot. Then I hate myself so much I have two or three slices of cake which I don't even fancy. Anyway, I was thrilled to be chosen to test this diet, and even more thrilled to say that I ate quite normally – which for me seemed a lot – and I even lost two pounds in the five days. I think it's marvellous.'

Anita Frame, forty-three, a dental receptionist, is a divorced mother of four

'I am very particular about how I look, especially as I've joined a dating agency recently and am going out on dates now. I needed to tone up a bit and probably should lose about a stone.

'On my other diets, if I went out I was terrified of having a pat of butter with my bread and I'd ask for any sauce to be left off. On this diet I felt completely liberated! It is difficult to describe, but I now just say yes to everything. As I have learnt to eat dainty amounts and not to worry that I'll never eat a square meal again, I feel as if all the tension of a diet has gone. I've done the programme now for three weeks and have lost half a stone, and the best thing is that I feel I'm not on a diet at all.

'I invited one man I met over to my house and cooked him the spaghetti with smoked salmon and dill. It took me about ten minutes from start to finish, and he was going mad, saying how fantastic it was and that I must have been slaving away for hours.
I didn't say anything!

'I just can't believe how toned I feel, and how flat my stomach is. I was really, really unsure of it when I was chosen, but now I'm telling all my friends about the Grenfell 5-Day programme. My children can all eat exactly the same as me, and as one of my daughters has quite a weight problem I'm pleased that she's losing weight too.'

Helen Foster, thirty-one, a unit-trust dealer, lives with her partner

'My porridge breakfast filled me up so much I almost didn't need my mid-morning snack every day, but I ate it and wasn't so hungry by lunchtime.

'I haven't much of a weight problem, but I'm always holding my stomach in. I didn't think I'd get used to the amount of food – usually I tend to pig out when I get home from work as I'm so hungry, but eating a mid-afternoon snack put paid to that. I could happily go right through until dinner and eat far less.

'I work at home these days, so I got a kitchen timer and put that to go off every hour. I just got on the floor and did twenty sit-ups. It sounds stupid, but it worked for me. I think they made all the difference.

'By day five I was definitely into the swing of it. At first, I thought I would be hungry, especially at night, but it seems that I am eating most of the time and I lost three pounds (1.4kg) by day four. I'm sure I've lost about one inch (2.5cm) off my hips! On day five I put on a skirt that I always use for testing my size and it felt quite roomy! Great!

'I'm starting the Lifetime Maintenance programme next week. I'm off on my holiday and I'll want to have a few drinks and sweet things but not undo all the good work I've just done. Then when I come back I will start the 5-Day programme again, in case I've gained any weight.

I know I do not have a real figure problem, but my stomach drives me mad and I'm always hiding it. This programme is just wonderful; I think I'll stay on it for good.'

Marian Crawford, thirty-seven, is a housewife with three children

'I'm tall, 5 foot 10 (1m 78cm), and I was stick-thin before I had the children. It's my stomach that gets me down, I feel I can take in tucks at the sides! Having children has been like blowing up a balloon, keeping it there all Christmas and letting it down again – it never goes back to what it was before, does it?

'I needed to tone up, and I found the best help were the stomach exercises. I've also got terrible insides. I'm on the go all day with the children and two new little puppies and I don't often eat much from breakfast to teatime. I was taking vitamins because I was tired, then laxatives because I was constipated! On this diet, I managed to give all that up. My stomach was less grumbly and felt much flatter, and I am pleased I don't have all that bloatedness now.

'I never used to drink much water or eat much fruit, and now I will, as it has sorted my problems out. I looked at the diet sheet and thought, "There's so much food – I'll put on weight", but I lost four pounds (1.8kg) and wasn't hungry for a minute. I'll definitely keep it up.'

Janet and Simon Ashworth, fifty-one and fifty, are both nurses at a Nottingham hospital and have grown-up children

Janet: 'We decided to go on the diet together, for support. Simon wouldn't have gone on any of my other diets (which I'm always starting!) because he says the food's too finicky, but when he saw omelettes, mashed potatoes and roast chicken his eyes lit up.

'I must admit I was a bit sceptical about adding crème fraiche to one dish and cooking something else in butter, but after all the years I've been on these low-fat spreads, good old butter was fantastic. I know you can't have lashings of it, but somehow knowing that you're eating the real thing makes you go easy on it anyway. It was like pure gold!

'I suppose I'm quite overweight – about two and a half stone – and Simon's the same. I've been dieting for as long as I can remember, but what puts me off is calculating the portions, measuring each out and then piling on

the vegetables because you can't eat again for hours. This diet was such common sense because you just eat small amounts of everything.

'My dress is much looser round my stomach, and I reckon to have lost two inches, although I can't have, can I? I'm going onto the Maintenance programme to lose the rest of my excess weight.'

Simon: 'I joined Janet to support her, thinking I'd hate it. In fact, I've lost weight too. I feel much, much smaller in my abdomen, and far brighter and healthier. I don't know what it is, but I'm really bouncing around now. I've managed to give up my morning chocolate bar with no cravings, and no diet's ever got me to do that!

'My favourite meal was the Coconut Chicken Curry. I wasn't sure about this while I was making it, but it tasted lovely.

'It was hard at first, I'll admit, to look at a small saucer of salad or a couple of spoons of veggies, but you soon want much less. I tried to eat a piece of fish and three potatoes today and had to stop after two of them, I was so full. I think this diet's the best thing that's ever happened to us.'

Louise Cordas, twenty-seven, is married with one child and another on the way

'I actually lost four stone (25.4kg) to get married! Then I put it back on, got pregnant and thought there wasn't any point. After Matthew was born I knew I should diet, but in the back of my mind was the thought that I knew we wanted two children quite close together and there wouldn't be any point in dieting only to get pregnant again.

'I started the diet just before I fell pregnant with this one, so obviously I've given it up for a bit, but I'll start it straight away after the birth. I totally believe in this diet. The main thing I like is that I can give my little boy anything I have to eat, which isn't the case with some fancy diet books with all their exotic menus. I never felt hungry, but I knew that if I did I could eat some yoghurt and not even think about it. I loved the pasta primavera. The pesto sauce with the crème fraiche was completely yummy, and it only took a few minutes. All the ingredients were in the local supermarket, so I got everything there and didn't have to traipse around.

'I can't wait to go back on it and lose all this weight again.'

Dee Whittaker, forty-eight, a beauty therapist, is widowed with two adult daughters

'Although I'm a beauty therapist, I've let myself go since my husband died. I always used to play badminton and swim, but the exercise went out of the window last year when I felt so depressed. My weight soared and I couldn't do anything about it.

'I've lost four pounds (1.8kg) and feel about a stone lighter. I actually found the posture section most revealing – I didn't realize until I caught sight of myself in a shop window that I was slouching so badly. My neck was all scrunched up and my chest seemed to sink into my stomach! I think about it all the time now, and it's made my stomach hold itself in and look controlled, which has made me look more confident, my friend tells me.

'I thought that exercising several times a day would be a chore, but I started to look forward to it. It was like sending myself on a course. I felt I had homework to do several times a day. Each page of the diet was like Monica talking to me and encouraging me, and the best encouragement was that she said it had worked for her.

'I don't want to stop. I feel I can adapt the ideas for myself now, which is the idea of the Maintenance pro- gramme. It starts off seeming weird with all that mashed potato, rice pudding and bananas, and I didn't think I'd like bio yoghurt. I'd recommend this diet plan to anyone of any age. My stomach's much, much flatter, and I've got my confidence back.'

Sally Pallister, twenty-three, is single and works as a journalist for a women's magazine

'My life is one mad rush from the beginning of the day to the end, and I go for long hours without eating. Then when I do, it's all the wrong things. I grab a sandwich or stop at one of the local bistros for a snack, which is usually a burger or curry, then I feel completely blown up for hours. I also sit at my computer for up to six hours without a break, and my bottom was spreading. I weighed about ten pounds (4.5kg) too much and my figure was a disgrace for someone my age, but I thought, "What can I do?"

'If I hadn't been chosen to be a tester I wouldn't have bothered with a diet, but when I saw the meals all written out for me it took away the responsibility and I said yes straight away. I'm so glad I did.

'What I liked was the simplicity. I'm always out, and my new cooker which I've had for six months is still in its cello- phane! I haven't got a freezer either, so it would have been no good if I'd needed frozen stuff. The food was the type anyone would like, with no preparation if you didn't want to, and it really worked. After the five days I was four pounds (1.8kg) lighter, but I felt really quite svelte. My stomach had lost all its hugeness and I didn't need to hold it in all the time. I did do the exercises too, which was an effort for me as I hate exercise, but as it was only a few minutes here and there I thought it was worth it. Frankly, I didn't think so few exercises would make a difference, but they have.

'I've decided to stick with the 5-Day plan every Monday to Friday and as I have a hectic social life at weekends I'll do my own thing then, though I won't go overboard. I'd recommend the diet to any of my friends.'

Molly Agnew, seventy-eight, is a retired headmistress

'I've always been careful about my appearance, and just because I'm retired it doesn't mean I've given up. I still like to wear tailored clothes and I have a lot of Christmas engagements this year.

'My stomach's more delicate than it used to be and I can't take too many spices or fibre. But the diet worked a treat. The starch was somehow calming and I've just worn a skirt I haven't fitted into for ten years!'

Linda Thompson, forty, an assistant recruitment manager in the NHS, is married with two children

'I'm a lifelong member of the diet club, and at the moment I'd say my weight's stable. I lost three pounds (1.4kg) on the diet, and my friend who did it with me lost a good inch off her stomach in only five days!

'I really liked the fact that when I started work at 9 a.m. I knew I didn't have to wait long before I could have a snack. I couldn't have gone on until lunchtime.

'We eat late in the evening at home, so I saved the main meal until 9 p.m. I particularly liked the fish content of the diet and I would definitely stick with the Maintenance plan. I think it was a great diet, and it was nice to see results so quickly. I never knew there were so many additives in the diet foods I'd been eating – it really makes you think, doesn't it?'

getting
down to it

Why Is Your Stomach So Big?

It does not take a medical degree to work out why your midsection
has got out of control:

1 you are constantly bloated

2 you are overweight

3 you are constipated

4 your muscles need toning

5 your posture is terrible

Before you feel too overwhelmed about yourself, let us look at each of
these in turn, and see how the Grenfell 5-Day programme can help:

1 You Are Constantly Bloated

This topic is really a book in itself. Has bloating always been a problem or is it worse these days? If it *has* got worse, do we know why? Did our grandparents suffer from bloated stomachs? And what does the term mean anyway?

By way of clearing the decks, I asked a gastroenterologist what was meant by bloating. It is most commonly intestinal gas, which causes pressure and distension of the abdomen. Women complain of it more than men do, but on investigation it was usually found that the amount of intestinal gas was the same in both sexes – women simply felt worse about it and had lower tolerance to it.

Our grandparents might well have experienced this sort of discomfort, but were accustomed to it. We are more sensitive these days, and certainly years ago people did not assume that gas, flatulence and wind were in any way unusual. Added to this is the fact that women wore corsets or foundation garments that held everything in place so a distended stomach could be hidden. I am not talking about the Dark Ages by the way. I was handed a small stretchy thing called a 'roll-on' as soon as I reached adolescence, its purpose being to hold in my young-womanly tummy. It was assumed that you needed one!

Hormonal shifts do make us feel bloated. The hormone oestrogen rises in mid-cycle as the lining of your womb prepares for a fertilized egg, and it has violent and sudden shifts when you are on the Change. This can make you feel full and uncomfortable. I have talked about this problem and given some real solutions in my book *Beat Your Body Chaos*, but as hormonal bloating is automatically resolved after a few days, I will not expound the subject here.

High-fibre products

Whole grains are wonderful and every diet should have them. However, they are sources of insoluble fibre – fibre that passes through the gut whole. Bran, the outer husk of grain, which acts as nature's 'scrubbing brush' can cause irritation to the gut, and the bacteria it produces in the large bowel ferment and produce gas. I suggest you avoid these altogether on your important days. You can either do the 5-Day programme any time you have something important coming along, or adopt it for just twenty-four hours simply by omitting all high-fibre foods.

Insoluble fibre is also found in:

• nuts

• rice

• strawberries

• many breakfast cereals.

Fruit

All fruit contains fructose (a form of carbohydrate) and it appears that most people have a limit to the amount of fructose they can absorb. When this limit is exceeded, fructose enters the colon, where it ferments, producing gas.

Some fruits also contain sorbitol, which is a natural sugar alcohol. Sorbitol-containing fruits seem to produce more gas than other fruits. Fruits containing sorbitol include:

• apples

• pears

• cherries

• plums

• peaches.

The juice of these fruits also contains sorbitol.

From a practical point of view, it makes sense to cut back on fruit if you suffer from a lot of gas. Do not eliminate fruit, but watch portion size. On the Grenfell programme, I encourage you to eat fruit in the evening to get maximum benefit from its laxative properties.

However, the reason some fruits are not suitable for those in search of a flat stomach is their fibre content. Apples have a lovely soluble fibre (see page 26) called pectin in their flesh – but their skin is insoluble fibre and will pass through your body as it came in. *All fruit skins can be a problem, so peel that fruit!* Though you must eat some skins if you become debilitatingly constipated.

Cruciferous vegetables

Cruciferous vegetables are a family of vegetables that includes cabbage, Brussels sprouts, cauliflower, broccoli and kale. You do not need me to tell you that these can cause a great deal of gas, so you will not eat them at all when you are doing the 5-Day programme.

Of course, when you are 'between programmes' or at any other time to suit yourself, feel free to eat as many of these wonderful vegetables as you like.

Pulses

Pulses include peas, all kinds of beans, lentils and sweetcorn. Pulses contain protein, they are low in fat and high in fibre because the outer skin or shell cannot be broken down by the body, so it passes through the system whole.

The reputation of beans and lentils as gas producers goes before them. It is said that if you eat them often enough, the effect ceases. Frankly, I would rather not take the risk!

Fizzy drinks

Do not have them! They are full of gas that simply passes through to your insides!

Food Intolerances

Irritable bowel syndrome (IBS) and food intolerances in general have been big news for the last few years. I am astounded that they have taken such a hold when one never used to hear of them. I can vaguely remember an aunt saying that cucumber 'didn't agree with her' or my mother complaining that coffee gave her heartburn, but that was it. Being intolerant of food was not a concept anyone would have recognized, unless of course they were seriously ill or suffering from a major food allergy. Coeliac disease, extreme hypersensitivity to gluten (found in wheat, oats, barley and rye), was also well documented. But sensitivity to bananas, bread or fish?

I am sure many people will dispute this. There are always exceptions to a rule and somebody will have suffered intolerances fifty years ago. Nonetheless, I go back to what I have just said: perfectly healthy, functioning adults would not have phoned before a dinner party to say they could not eat wheat or dairy foods, neither would they demand that a restaurant adapt their meals to accommodate their food intolerances. Not if they were otherwise healthy. The 'done' thing was to shift the food round your plate, eat what you could manage and disguise what you had left under a few vegetables. We have all struggled through a plate of something disgusting swimming in grease, but that's life.

This diet makes much of foods to avoid or leave for another time, but this is a trick to help you achieve the best results. I am not suggesting that you have an intolerance simply because some foods tend to make you flatulent, constipated or bloated.

When you read the next section, about chemicals and additives, you will see what I mean. I certainly believe that what we eat can cause havoc in our insides, but that is due to the massive amounts of chemicals added. When you read my directions on eating, swallowing, chewing and so on, you will see that eating habits are another questionable area. Poor eating habits can have the most devastating effects on

your system, including foul gas, bloating, excess acid and a feeling of fullness hours after a meal. It is no wonder that you immediately blame what you have just eaten, and as wheat is in so many foods, and is eaten in some form or another for breakfast (cereal, toast), lunch (sandwiches) and snacks (biscuits, cake), it is not surprising that wheat is a contender when we look for something to blame.

But who eats 'wheat'? Bread has other things in it, a sandwich has a filling, pasta and pizzas have toppings, and what about the salads that come on the side or the fruit juice you drank after your breakfast toast?

In other words, wheat alone may not be to blame.

I would look instead to soya flour and to emulsifiers. Soya, while perfectly good and nutritious, can be an allergen. It can cause a mild reaction in some people, who will probably not even know that they have a sensitivity to it. Personally, I stay a million miles from anything with soya, not because I am allergic but because I dislike the inevitable effects. It has a tendency – I will put it no stronger than that – to cause bloating.

Then there are emulsifiers. Look at the wrapping on a standard loaf of commercial bread and I bet you will see these listed along with the soya. There are other things too, and often the loaves are treated to make them last a week or even two. If your loaf is still fresh after a week, avoid it next time. Proper bread should be stale after a couple of days.

My answer is to make your own bread. A recipe for this is on page 114. It might seem fiddly, but if you make several loaves you can slice and freeze them, ready to take slices as you need them. You also have the satisfaction of eating your own wholesome bread, free from soya flour and artificial additives.

I would be foolish to suggest that food intolerances do not exist. Of course they do. But please try my simple practical measures before dismissing whole food groups from your diet.

Let me read to you the list of ingredients from a standard pack of own-brand white rolls from a leading supermarket:

Wheat flour, Water, Vegetable oil, Hydrogenated vegetable oil, Salt, Yeast, Dextrose, Emulsifiers: Sodium stearyl-2-lactylate and Mono- and diacetyl tartaric acid; Esters of mono- and diglycerides of fatty acids, Soya flour, Flour treatment agent: L-ascorbic acid

The pack also states that the rolls 'may contain traces of nuts and sesame seeds'.

Now, I have been making my own bread for years, and to make white bread I use unbleached wheat flour, yeast, water, salt, sugar and a little butter or olive oil. Nothing else. The bread keeps a couple of days; if I want to keep it longer, I freeze it.

I am still struggling to understand why bought bread needs all those extra ingredients. I found similar ingredients in cereal bars, cakes, soups, packet sauces and so on. The lists would take several pages of this book. The real question is: what are all these additives doing to your body?

The additives are harmless. They would not be there if they weren't. But I truly believe it has been forgotten that our bodies were designed to process food and water. We are incredibly robust and, with a good amount of stomach acid, thorough chewing and a stable environment (which means not too much stress), our digestive system can tackle most things. But emulsifiers? Hydrogenated fat, which is known to be a health risk? And while I am at it, what are traces of nuts and sesame seeds doing in white bread?

Additives are thought of as essential because without them our food spoils more quickly. They prevent hardness and rancidity, and in many cases additives inhibit the growth of salmonella and other harmful bacteria. It would be wrong to condemn them out of hand, but few people realize that many additives cause the discomfort of abdominal bloating and wind, and the distended stomach we simply can't hold in.

In the quest for a lower-fat diet, manufacturers have had to come up with increasingly creative ways of cutting calories in their products without sacrificing the taste. They have found that adding seaweeds, gums and emulsifiers, not to mention pumping vast quantities of air into everything, makes low-calorie food look and taste like the real thing. The drawbacks have been twofold: first, you tend to eat twice as much because you think you are getting half the calories, and second, the additives have unfortunate effects on your digestive system.

Don't get me wrong. I am not a health freak. I just don't see the point in the tiny calorie saving if the results are unflattering and embarrassing.

Here is a list of the most commonly used additives which have a laxative effect, and therefore cause a grumbling and flatulent stomach:

Sorbitol (E420), isomalt, mannitol and xylitol

These are all sweeteners known to have a laxative effect in high doses. Found in sausages, soft-scoop ice cream, diabetic jams and sugar-free sweets. In susceptible individuals, especially children, the effects can include a distressingly distended stomach.

Sorbitol is also present quite naturally in fruits like apples, cherries, peaches, apricots and plums, and these fruits seem to produce more gas than other fruits do.

Carrageenan (E407)

This seaweed-derived product is an emulsifier, and is used to thicken and improve consistency. Found in quick-setting jellies, milkshakes, biscuits, pastries, meat pies, sausages and instant mousses. Has caused concern for its laxative effect, especially in children.

Guar gum (E412), gum arabic (E414) and xanthan gum (E415)

Can cause flatulence through a laxative effect. Found in salad creams, meringue mixes, salad dressings, soft cheese, coleslaw, canned vegetables, processed cheese, pickles, fruit gums, wine, beer, confectionery and yoghurts.

Air

Not an additive in the accepted sense, but included here because it is added to some foods to give them volume. For example, ice creams and dessert mousses are often pumped with air to lower the calorie content weight for weight. Taking in extra air is the primary cause of intestinal wind, so avoid foods which boast very low calories if possible.

The list of lesser-known and little-used additives which can cause intestinal problems is long, but they need not concern us here as my object is to alert you to the most commonly used additives that you are likely to find in your everyday foods. I must stress that these substances are not harmful in small doses, but remember that the average diet – especially a slimming diet – will probably include not just one or two, but many of these products every day. The cumulative laxative effect of these additives is something you are unlikely to be aware of. Personally, I see little virtue in giving up natural sugar only to eat large quantities of chemical alternatives.

I am not including a comprehensive discussion of additives because I believe the solution is obvious – eat fresh food. The Grenfell 5-Day programme uses only fresh ingredients to make meals that are easy to prepare and even easier to freeze, so if you want convenience food, you can have home-cooked, additive-free meals to hand at any time.

Next on the list of causes of bloating is how you eat. This is one of the most important factors, and the point where I start to sound like a mother telling off her children for not minding their table manners! Even if you eliminate the wrong foods, all your good intentions will be thwarted if you eat the wrong way. Being on the programme means you have to be rigid about how you eat.

Eat slowly

When you see food and smell it, your digestive juices start flowing. This is stomach acid, ready to break down your food and churn it into a paste before sending it on its way through your gut. If you see food and gulp it down, huge lumps of food enter the stomach, which has to grind away on overtime to turn it into something manageable. The result: gas!

Another cause of intestinal wind is swallowed air. You swallow air when you:

- talk or laugh while eating

- chew gum

- slurp drinks

- slurp food

- take too much food onto your fork – you know it's too much when it is hard to fit it all in your mouth!

The result is great pockets of air that blow you out.

It's hard to train yourself to eat slowly, especially if you were brought up in a household where everyone ate as fast as possible, or if you missed out on second helpings if you ate too slowly. It's hard if you have only a short time in which to eat. But if you eat more slowly and carefully you will feel full much sooner, and this way you will eat less.

Chew food to a paste

A typical food-bolter is usually loading the fork or spoon before the previous mouthful has been swallowed. This is a bad habit. Train yourself to put your cutlery down between mouthfuls and not pick it up again until you have swallowed. The digestive system works to a series of signals, the first of which is the chewing action. This alerts your system that something is on its way and stomach acids are set in motion. The longer you chew, the more acid is produced and, of course, the food is then nicely broken up, can be digested with the minimum of fuss and you feel fine.

Chewing something once or twice before swallowing does not allow your stomach to get ready. It also has to deal with lumps of food rather than a nice paste. Chewing will go a long way to *significantly* reducing bloating.

Try not to eat under stress

Easier said than done, but if a problem is gnawing away at you, or you are sitting at the dinner table fuming after an argument, the effects on your digestion can be pretty unpleasant. The most common complaint is painful stomach cramps an hour or two after eating. An attack of nerves, such as on an important date or before an interview, can also bring on the most dreadful spasms. If you are under stress during a meal, avoid meat and poultry and stick with fish and mashed root vegetables like parsnip, potatoes and carrots.

Do not leave long gaps between meals

Leaving more than three hours between small meals means that you not only get hungry and are therefore likely to eat more than you need, but also that the build-up of stomach acid and emptiness can lead to indigestion. Think in terms of a yawning, empty hole in your stomach which suddenly receives a massive amount of food all at once, and probably too quickly. Being on a diet that restricts you to only three meals a day means that you will tend to make the most of every meal. Your stomach, which has been empty for up to five waking hours, then has to cope with a lot of food in one go. If you have a bloating problem, you should not go for more than three hours during the day without something in your stomach.

2 You Are Overweight

Fat settles all too easily on your stomach. This is because the midsection gets the least movement. Everyday routine forces us to move our arms and legs, but the midsection needs specific movements. Sitting for hours on end is the real killer. But even if you get up and get moving and get a good fat-loss diet going, you could still fail to crack this problem. This is because the key is not what you eat, but why you eat.

Eating when bored

You might not feel bored as you rush around with ten things to do at once, but you can be bored of being busy. Food becomes a time-filler.

So don't fill time with eating! There are so many other productive things to do. If your place is a tip, clear out a drawer. Tidy a room. Rather than eat, take the fridge apart and enjoy chucking out leftovers. You will have the benefits of a job done as well as the saving of your waistline.

Eating the wrong things

There's no such thing as a bad food. Not even chocolate or chips or sugar or butter. There are only bad diets. Eating chocolate is not a problem and chips are not fattening. What *is* wrong is a diet of chips, then chocolate, followed by lots of alcohol. Day after day! A balance of small amounts of everything is the key to a great body and flat stomach.

Not using up your food intake

Fat settles because your food is surplus to requirements. Nothing very earth-shattering there. So why not make your requirements greater? Exercise doesn't have to be manic fitness; it can be movement of any kind. Each time you move, you raise your calorie-burn rate slightly. If you move fast, you raise it more. If you put in a bit more effort, like going from walking on the flat to climbing stairs, the calorie-burn rises again, taking you from one calorie a minute burned to four calories a minute, and so on. This is a terrific way to increase calorie requirements rather than eating less.

Metabolic rates and eating too little

If you lay in bed doing absolutely nothing all day, you would still need energy to keep you alive. This is called your Basal Metabolic Rate (BMR). In fact, you can work out your BMR – how much energy your body uses up just keeping you alive – like this:

For women	For men
weight in kg x 2 x 11	weight in kg x 2 x 12

So, for a woman weighing 55kg: BMR $= 55 \times 2 \times 11 = 110 \times 11 = 1,210$ calories.

To work out your actual energy requirements, you have to take your lifestyle into account.

- If you are sedentary, multiply your BMR by 120 (so the 55kg woman taking little exercise would require 1,210 calories x 120 = 1,452 calories per day)

- If you are fairly active (you walk two or three times a week): BMR x 130

- If you are moderately active (you exercise two or three times a week): BMR x 140

- If you are very active (hard exercise four or more times a week): BMR x 150

Eating too little actually makes you gain weight in the long run. Your body is programmed to preserve life, so if your food intake is reduced your metabolism slows down. It doesn't happen overnight. If you remember that nature's job is to preserve life at all costs, you can understand why cutting out food in order to stay slim just does not work. If you have consistently irregular eating patterns, your metabolism will slow down to preserve your fat supplies as your body adjusts to try to keep you alive as long as possible. Eating little and often serves the dual purpose of preventing weight gain and keeping your metabolism ticking away happily at a moderate rate, so that the calories you have taken in are burnt efficiently.

Lack of will power

You might say you lack will power. This is an easy cop-out to save your brain from having to exert any reasonable psychological force. Lack of will power happens when you see a diet as something unpleasant and avoidable. But isn't getting up night after night to a crying baby unpleasant? Or going to do a job you don't like every day? But you would do it, and this proves that you *do* have will power in some form.

The Grenfell programme is a daily reminder of the things you have to do because they become part of your life. Rather than being on a diet, you are on a programme that will fit beautifully into your life. You won't lack will power ever again.

Beating Cravings

The greater the distance between wanting something and having it, the less likely you are to end up with it. This is how credit cards work. If you had to go home and get the cash every time you saw a fabulous outfit, you would only buy a fraction of what you see. A credit card turns wanting into having all too quickly, and this is how cravings take hold.

If you fancy chocolate when chocolate is in the cupboard – well, you know the outcome. Not to succumb would be torment. One way to beat the cravings is to put as much distance as possible between you and the food. In other words, don't buy it.

Secondly, remember that cravings go. It is impossible to sustain desire, as anybody who has given up cigarettes will tell you. I gave up cigarettes. At first, you have to learn a completely new agenda for what to do in the times when you used to have a cigarette. You have to think yourself into a whole new person. What do non-smokers do? But after a few months things are not so bad and after a year you don't crave cigarettes at all. After ten years, I can tell you, you don't even think about them. Surely if you were hooked on cigarettes, it was impossible to do without them. Obviously not.

The same applies to food cravings. You cannot go without food, but you can give up things that are bad for you. Beating cravings means giving up completely, at least until you have got that habit or that food out of your system. That is why I never allow 'treats' of junk food or sweets on any of my diets. It is like offering an alcoholic a drink as a treat. You just wouldn't do it.

The 5-Day programme banishes bad foods, but the Maintenance programme does too. I'm not going to pretend that there is some weird and wonderful method for dealing with cravings. Why make life difficult for yourself by keeping the objects of your temptation around to torture you? You have to be strict, give them up and never look back. This is for your own good!

Allowing some 'unlimited' foods

This is another tricky area. People always want to find some food in a diet that is 'unlimited'. This to say that if you want more to eat, there is some food with which you can pile your plate as high as you like. Well, I am afraid I call this gluttony. If you are serious about learning new eating habits, unlimited food has to go. Even nibbling on raw carrots. If you have a problem with food, you must learn to eat smaller, daintier meals. On my diet, nothing is unlimited.

This is not to say that I blame you. In my house as a child there was a policy of eating everything on the plate. We had healthy eating habits, but my mother could whip up a Victoria sponge filled with fresh cream in no time, and we were encouraged to eat as much of this healthy, 'natural' cake as possible. I never put on what we would call 'weight' in those days, because the culture was that if you gained half a stone, you made sure you lost it pretty fast. However, controlling my gargantuan appetite was a challenge and I managed it by pretending to be a film star who toyed with tiny, stylish portions. This was another trick that gave me a flat stomach, and it works.

If you have a big appetite and no weight problem, you can have any unlimited food you like. But if you are overweight and yearn for a flatter stomach, you have to meet me halfway and give up the nibbling. Don't have unlimited amounts of food. Think stylish, and get your appetite down.

3 You Are Constipated

If there is anything worse than food going through you too quickly, it is food going through too slowly! You feel full-up and you look it. Constipation can be caused by:

- eating too much meat
- eating a high protein diet generally
- drinking too much tea
- eating too little fibre
- not drinking enough water
- some iron tablets
- some anti-depressant drugs.

Long-term use of laxatives can be extremely harmful to your body, as they prevent it from functioning in its own natural way and the end result is a lazy gut. They also cause a lot of fluid to be lost from the body, which you aren't aware of until you have a blinding headache.

People used to shovel down massive quantities of fibre because they believed it was healthy. It is, but it is also irritating to the stomach and this is what it is meant to be. Dealing with constipation – and I am all too aware that this is hardly an elegant topic – is easily done on your 5-Day programme by having what is in effect a laxative evening meal or supper. All those vegetables which you couldn't eat during the day, like sweetcorn and broad beans, can now be eaten with abandon, and my recommended nightly dessert of prunes and half-fat crème fraiche is a treat you have to look forward to!

The last two causes of a big stomach, poorly toned muscles and bad posture, are dealt with in the section 'Exercise and Posture'.

A Quick Guide to Nutrition

A common misconception is that if you want a healthy, nutritious diet, you have to spend a fortune on fancy, gourmet foods. In fact, as long as you satisfy your body's needs for the right balance of carbohydrates, proteins and fats, you needn't spend more than a few pounds a week, a lot less than you would if you constantly snacked on chocolate and ate takeaways.

My diet is particularly satisfying because there are no long periods without food. It does not have a huge amount of bulk, but it is quite high in carbohydrates – the foods that supply ready energy.

Carbohydrates

If you are stuck for a definition of a carbohydrate, think of anything that was a leaf, root, fruit, seed, nut, or grain. Plants, in other words. Even a simple spinach leaf has carbohydrate in it.

Carbohydrates fall into two categories: simple and complex.

They come in three main forms: sugars, starch and fibre.

Simple carbohydrates are sugars:

- lactose is found in milk and dairy products and is half as sweet as sugar

- glucose is found in vegetables, fruit and honey

- sucrose is found in fruit and vegetables

- fructose is found in fruit and honey

- maltose is found in malt extract, barley, grains and malted wheat.

Complex carbohydrates include starches found in bread, potatoes, rice, pasta, cereals and nuts, as well as fibres found in unrefined foods

Most carbohydrates are broken down during digestion. Although insoluble fibre is not digested, it nourishes bacteria in the large bowel and there is subsequent fermentation – need I say more?

However, do not exclude fibre for good. There is another type of fibre called soluble fibre, which is more easily absorbed by the gut and which is found in the following foods:

- breakfast oats

- fruit

- vegetables.

Soluble fibre has many health benefits and is included in your 5-Day programme. It helps reduce cholesterol in the blood and also slows the absorption of glucose, preventing sudden rises in blood sugar – particularly useful for diabetics.

Be wary of resistant starch. This is a type of starch that cannot be broken down by enzymes in the small intestine in the normal way. It is found in raw potatoes, unripe fruit and some processed foods. It passes undigested into the large intestine where it can ferment, causing wind and extreme discomfort. You have been warned!

A high-carbohydrate diet replenishes and increases the body's reserves of glycogens, which play an important role in providing a readily usable energy supply and making you feel lively. A common complaint of dieters over the years has been the tiredness that almost inevitably accompanies low-calorie diets, but by eating the correct balance of proteins, carbohydrates and fats you should be able to lose weight steadily, and with no ill effects.

Proteins

Although only about twenty per cent of our daily nutritional requirements are for protein, every cell in the human body needs it. Without it, tissue cannot be repaired effectively, nor can new cells grow. If you starve yourself on diets that give you hardly anything to eat, you are also doing a disservice to your looks. Proteins such as keratin and collagen keep your skin supple and young-looking and your hair strong and elastic. Protein also helps fight infection and aids digestion.

You will be nourished by a good balance of proteins on this diet.

Proteins come from two sources: plants and animals.

Animal proteins		Plant proteins	
cheese	fish	wheat	beans
meat	poultry	bread	potatoes
milk	eggs	rice	nuts

Proteins cannot be stored by the body. Excess proteins are converted to glucose by the liver. If your diet is too rich in protein – for example, if you eat a lot of cheese or meat, you run the risk of osteoporosis because, strange as it may seem when you are eating calcium from cheese, too much protein can result in loss of calcium.

On the 5-Day programme you will be eating most of the proteins listed above, with the exception of beans, and with only a very small amount of nuts, of which you need only a small quantity anyway. Just two Brazil nuts every day provide the average body with all it needs of some minerals, such as selenium, and also provide useful amounts of fat. A simple bowl of cereal with milk provides roughly one third of our daily recommended protein intake, so it is unlikely that many of us are deficient in protein.

Fats

Fat is essential. Without it, vitamins A, D and E cannot be absorbed from the gut and you can become severely vitamin-deficient, leading to illness. Fats form every membrane in every cell of the human body. It is vital that you do not exclude fat from your everyday meals.

Like proteins, fats also come from two sources: plant and animal. The 'fat issue' is often a source of worry and topic of conversation, and ignorance is usually the cause. So here is a simple breakdown of the types of fat in our foods.

Animal fats
These are the so-called bad fats, found in:

- dairy foods

- milk

- meat.

In fact, all these foods were also in our list of proteins. The saturated fat (see below) contained in these foods is considered to be bad for the health of your heart. A rule of thumb is that if the fat is the type that solidifies when cooled after heating (like lard), it is less good for you.

Vegetable fats
Vegetable fats are mainly oils like olive oil, sunflower oil and oil from nuts which contain a high proportion of unsaturated fatty acids (see below). They are generally thought to be better for health, although this is irrelevant when considering the question of weight loss, as all fats contain the same number of calories per ounce.

Saturated and unsaturated
Fats are made up of fatty acids. The two main types of fats are saturated and unsaturated. Saturated fats are solid at room temperature –like butter – and are found in most animal products, such as eggs, milk and meat. Unsaturated fats are liquid, like sunflower oil. The unsaturated fats are then divided into monounsaturated

and polyunsaturated. Saturated and monounsaturated fatty acids can be manufactured by the body from carbohydrates, alcohol and protein, so it is not essential to take extra supplies. Sources of monounsaturated fats include avocados, nuts, seeds, olive oil and fish oils.

Some polyunsaturated fatty acids cannot be made by the body and must therefore be taken in the form of the foods which contain them. These fatty acids are therefore called 'essential', and are made up of two groups called Omega-6 (found in vegetable oils) and Omega-3 (found in soya bean oil, rapeseed oil, oily fish, such as sardines, herrings, mackerel and salmon and the liver of white fish).

An adult requires about 4g of Omega-6 fatty acids a day (a handful of almonds or two teaspoons of sunflower oil) with a maximum of 25g. Very high intakes may be harmful. Omega-3 fatty acids are needed in small amounts: 1–2g a day (a handful of walnuts or a small portion of oily fish). Deficiency in either fatty acid can lead to poor growth, skin problems and a weakened immune system.

Transfats

Transfats are added to products to prevent them becoming hard and rancid. Look out for 'hydrogenated' on labels of foods such as margarine. They are found mainly in processed foods, such as crisps, cakes and biscuits.

On this diet you will not need to concern yourself with transfats as you won't be eating processed foods.

Fat is a necessary part of any good diet, but the key to healthy eating and weight loss is the percentage of your daily diet which fats make up. Experts disagree, but a sensible level would be no more than twenty per cent of your diet.

Vitamins and Minerals

Each individual will have different nutritional needs, but it is fair to say that guidelines can be set for the average man or woman who is in good health, regardless of occupation, age or size. The only adjustments which need to be taken into account are for very old people and young children, for pregnant and/or nursing mothers and for people engaged in particularly strenuous physical activity.

Vitamins are usually classed as water-soluble or fat-soluble. Water-soluble vitamins are all the B vitamins and vitamin C, and they cannot be stored by the body as any excess is excreted in the urine. Thus, a person who takes a massive amount of vitamin C each day in the hope that it will be stored to ward off a cold is wasting money. Never take too many vitamins, as they can be poisonous to the system. Always read the label on the bottle.

Vitamins A, D, E and K are fat-soluble, which means that they need an intake of fat to be absorbed. Unlike water-soluble vitamins, these are stored by the body which means that any excess can be extremely dangerous for your health.

Essential minerals

A balanced diet will also include adequate amounts of some trace elements and minerals, including calcium and iron, and it is important to know their sources.

Iron – sources include red meat, pulses, oatmeal, wholemeal bread, nuts, parsley, egg yolks and fortified breakfast cereals. Iron is lost through perspiration, so supplements might be needed if you exercise a lot.

Calcium – sources include milk and butter, cheese, nuts, sunflower seeds, soya products and leafy vegetables.

Folic acid – sources include leafy vegetables, beans, eggs, peanuts, fruit and wholegrain cereals.

Vegetarians and vegans, in particular, have need of non-meat sources of iron and vitamin B12.

Other minerals such as iodine and manganese, known as trace elements, are needed in tiny amounts, while potassium, sodium and magnesium are needed in quite large quantities. However, on this diet, you will be eating all you require of these minerals.

Vitamin supplements

Should you be taking vitamin or mineral supplements on this diet? Many people pop dozens of pills every day without the slightest idea of what they are taking or whether they need them. I don't take any supplements at all. That is not to say that I recommend everyone to stay supplement-free, and if you are a pregnant or nursing mother, have been ill or are elderly it might be good to check with your doctor that you are 100 per cent fit and healthy without supplements.

But do remember that supplements are exactly that. They are in addition to your food and not instead of it.

What most people don't realize, however, is that these nutrients are lost in different ways and at different rates according to our lifestyles, and no two people's needs are the same.

Stress and anxiety count for the loss of many nutrients from the body, as does an active lifestyle, so a very busy person could need extra vitamins and minerals. If you smoke, you lose 25mg ($^3/_4$oz) of vitamin C every time you light up. Cigarette smoking inhibits the absorption of vitamin C, as does the polluted atmosphere of an inner city, so if this is you, you'll need a supplement.

Coffee and tea drinking also inhibit absorption of vitamins, so if you drink a lot of these (more than four–six cups a day), either cut down, switch to the caffeine-free varieties or take extra vitamins. The small amount of vitamins you are losing may not seem much, but remember that the effect is cumulative. If you drink some caffeine, have the odd cigarette, drink alcohol daily, live in the city and have a pressured life, you are practically picking out tombstones! The point is, we can generally get away with it while we are young. We can smoke, drink and party all night, and still bounce out of bed in the morning looking fabulous. Wait a few years, though, and you'll have a different

tale to tell, and I know many dozens of women who speak of their past excesses with regret. You don't want to live like a hermit, but neither do you want to end up in a few years' time with a bad back and looking like a raddled old bag, all because you couldn't be bothered to take a bit of care.

It goes without saying that an active lifestyle demands more from your body. Keen exercisers need extra iron, as they lose iron through sweating, and of course strict slimmers should take a multivitamin and mineral supplement every day – or maybe not be such strict slimmers.

If you drink alcohol heavily, not only are you damaging your health through dehydration and liver toxicity, but you could be in danger of a deficiency of thiamine (vitamin B1) which is needed to convert carbohydrates and fats into energy. Symptoms include lethargy, muscle weakness and numbness.

As I have said, vitamin A in quantity can be toxic and extremely hazardous to health. Pregnant women should avoid eating liver for this reason, and should never take a vitamin A supplement due to possible damage to the unborn baby.

If you have been neglecting yourself this 5-Day plan will be a breath of fresh air. Because we all have different needs due to age and lifestyle, I suggest you get personalized advice on vitamin and mineral supplements. This programme, however, gives you all the nutrients you need.

The Diet

So What Am I Going To Eat?

I am pretty certain that your usual diet style is to race out enthusiastically and buy up half the supermarket. Your fridge is stuffed with chicken breasts and cottage cheese, fruit and colourful salad ingredients and this is surely all to the good. Well, is it? Maybe this preoccupation with food is what got you into this mess in the first place.

Learning about tasty, delicious and inventive ways with food is wonderful if you are happy with your weight. If you are reducing, it's not so good. Being preoccupied with food is like giving an alcoholic a job pulling pints. Why torture yourself?

Save your gourmet recipes for your Maintenance programme, for entertaining or for when you have lost the weight and got your tummy so deliciously flat you'll want to keep it that way. Never lapse on the 5-Day programme. Dealing with your tummy problem means simple food, splendidly presented, which takes hardly any time to make. I know you might have others to feed, but the great thing about my programme is that you can do your own thing during the day, when you might only have yourself to look after, and join everyone else in the evening for a good meal.

And simple food doesn't have to be boring. If you love elegant meals, serve food on your best tableware, if you have any, and sit down as if you were eating out. Smoked salmon, soufflés and herb omelettes are simple, but chic. Plain food is wonderful for your figure. So batten down the hatches for a few days and stock up on fish, eggs, avocados and fromage frais. This is going to be a proper diet.

The Rules – Start By Getting Strict

It is necessary that you take yourself in hand now, so keep to these golden rules.

DO

1 eat every three hours

2 drink water between meals

3 steer clear of starchy carbohydrates and high-fibre foods during the day

4 eat your fruit during the evening

5 stick to the portion-control rules – nothing is unlimited.

DO NOT

1 use artificial sweeteners

2 buy or eat any ready-meals or fast food

3 skip breakfast

4 go to bed hungry.

Your Guidelines for Eating

1 Do not put more on your plate than your portion allowances.

2 Try not to have second helpings.

3 Never load your fork or spoon with the next mouthful before you have swallowed the previous one.

4 If you feel full, stop eating. Put the plate aside and come back to it later.

5 Do not swallow your food until it is thoroughly chewed.

6 Where possible, as in the case of apples, slice food into manageable pieces rather than eat whole. Put on a plate and sit down to eat; this will encourage moderation.

I apologize if this sounds like a mother teaching her children table manners, but problems with food and weight often have their root cause in bad eating habits. Don't treat every meal as if you won't get the chance to eat ever again.

You do not have to go out and buy expensive foods like salmon and prawns if you do not wish to. You might not have a kitchen which is equipped for a lot of preparation and cooking, or you might live on your own and find making a whole dish just too complicated or time-consuming. However, the diet lasts only five days and is intended to produce results, so it's worth putting yourself out to get the recommended foods.

I have included a vegetarian recipe section and most of the pasta dishes are suitable for vegetarians, but I generally find that most vegetarians are expert at adapting ideas for their own tastes. Many of the recipes and menu choices are for use on the Maintenance programme only, of course.

What Will I Drink?

Sorry to be a party pooper. No alcohol is allowed on the 5-Day plan, but it won't kill you. When you progress to the Maintenance plan, you can have a couple of glasses of wine a day, lager or the odd glass of champagne, if you choose.

Try not to drink much water with your meal. It is fine to have a glass to hand, especially when you are with others as they might think it odd if you do not drink at all, but take small sips. Add a slice of fresh orange to make it taste different. It is important not to drink massive quantities of water with food because your stomach acids need to be strong for good digestion. Weak digestive juices mean your food will not be digested as robustly and this can lead to indigestion and feeling that your meal 'just hasn't gone down'.

Have plenty of water between meals. Aim to drink 2 litres (3½ pints) every day. In addition, drink tea and decaffeinated coffee as you wish. No fizzy drinks are allowed. Remember that they encourage gas in the intestines which can result in flatulence.

What If I Get Hungry?

I'll let you into a secret. I often have all-day photo-shoots dressed in a leotard and tight leggings. I have to stay in this garb for up to six hours and naturally I get hungry. But what about the flat stomach? I am doing exercise shots after all and it wouldn't do to find it hard to hold myself in!

I simply get a large tub of bio live yoghurt and keep it by the set. Every half hour or so I take another spoonful. It keeps me going brilliantly because it bathes the stomach so I don't feel hungry. And as you know by now, yoghurt has carbohydrate which gives me energy. It needs hardly any digesting, so it's like putting liquid into a food processor – no grinding or chopping. I keep my flat tummy and I end the day without one second of hunger.

Now, I am not suggesting that you live on yoghurt! But you'll find ways of compromising and sometimes you need liquids rather than solids to keep rumbles at bay. Thirst can feel like hunger. Have a drink of water or skimmed milk but *always wait to eat until your next scheduled meal*. Picking and snacking are terrible for waking up a nicely snoozing tummy and setting all that grinding off again.

Nearly There . . .

Before you get going, you need to get rid of the past. You are entering a new phase of your life – the newer, better version of yourself. You bear a striking resemblance to the old you, but you are not the same person. Act as if you are taking over this person's house after she has moved out and start by chucking out all her old rubbish.

1 Give away all those packets of dried fruit and tins of baked beans that are sitting at the back of your larder. Somebody will appreciate them.

2 Tell the family that you don't want bad food in the house. Insist they don't have it – you are in charge of what your children eat, after all. If you live with someone, you can still eat what they are having in the evening – just a bit less of it. This is not going to affect their meals at all.

3 Buy what you need – don't 'stock up'. This isn't a siege. Get a week's supply of foods like chicken, fish, avocados, fruits and vegetables, potatoes, pasta and rice. Buy plenty of bio yoghurt, cottage cheese, milk and oats.

4 Weigh yourself, take measurements and write them down here. I suggest:

Weight ....
Over bust under armpits ....
Bust line at fullest point ....
Under bust ....
Waist ....
Just below the navel ....
In line with the pubic bone ....
Hips at fullest point ....
Each thigh approximately six inches below top of legs
        left: .... right: ....
3 inches (7cm) above each knee
        left: .... right: ....
Each calf   left: .... right: ....
Each ankle left: .... right: ....

These measurements give you the best possible 'snapshot' of your figure. If fat is lost from the back (and this is often the second place to go – the first is the face) your bust measurement will be smaller. If you lose weight from your buttocks, your abdominal measurement will go down. If you tone up your buttocks you might find your abdomen feels tight. In addition, you can often *feel* fat and be convinced you have gained weight, or feel thin and think you can relax, but the gentle reminder of these few statistics will tell another story. I still have the measurements I wrote down in my 1977 diary – so I know where the fat has gone! Since then I have taken my measurements every January, which, I can tell you, makes fascinating reading. So please make a note of your statistics as well as your weight – there will be no excuse for not knowing if you have made progress!

BASIC RULES BEFORE YOU GET STARTED

- Eat breakfast within an hour of waking. If you are going to the gym or for a run, etc., and you won't be having breakfast until later, have a small snack like a few tablespoons of yoghurt, a glass of milk or two tablespoons of plain oats soaked in milk before you go.

- Eat from a 22cm (9-inch) dinner plate. Go and buy one if you don't have one already. This simply keeps portions small as you cannot actually pile more onto your plate. Do not have second helpings, either!

- Eat sitting down, at a table. Never spend less than ten minutes, preferably fifteen to twenty minutes, eating any one course.

- Measure portions by the tablespoon.

- Ban all foods sweetened with sorbitol or aspartame.

- Have plenty of water between meals. Aim to drink 2 litres (3½ pints) every day.

Recommended Foods

Plain, bio yoghurt

I cannot recommend 'bio' yoghurt highly enough. It is a complete food, meaning it contains all three main food groups: protein, carbohydrate and fat together. Few foods have them all. Your yoghurt should contain mildly fermented 'live' cultures of L-acidophilus, L. Casei and Bifidobacterium. Check the pot for information.

100g (3½oz) plain, bio yoghurt has approximately 4.2g protein, 3.5g fat and 5.3g carbohydrate.

Plain oats

Oats contain soluble fibre, which is extra kind to your insides. The carbohydrates help keep you full for longer, and the steady release of energy ensures you feel good and beat tiredness slumps.

30g (1oz) oats has 3.7g protein, 2.6g fat and 22g carbohydrate.

Fish

You can eat any fish! Kind to the gut, you may pan-fry it in butter, poach it in milk, grill or steam it. Other ways with fish are given in the recipe section, but suffice to say that you won't be bored with your fish.

150g (5oz) white fish has about 26g protein, 4.8g fat and a trace of carbohydrate.

150g (5oz) oily fish, such as salmon or mackerel, has 24–34g protein, 13–28g fat and no carbohydrate, although it is important to note that the fat is mostly monounsaturated and therefore healthy, and the saturated fat content is as low as 2–5g.

A small tin of tuna fish has around 25g protein, 8g fat and no carbohydrate.

100g (3½oz) shellfish, like prawns and crab, have 14g protein, almost no fat at 0.5g and no carbohydrate.

Eggs

Eggs are brilliant. It is probably because I have chickens at home, but I have always based my diet on eggs – not surprising when I only have to walk down to the nest box and collect a handful of freshly laid, nutritious eggs. And they're such powerhouses of goodness! I routinely hard-boil half a dozen to keep ready in my fridge from where I can slice and scatter them over a salad, slice onto crispbreads for a light meal, put into a sandwich or just eat whole.

A plate of scrambled or poached eggs or a three-egg omelette has 19g protein, 5.4g fat and no carbohydrate.

Leafy greens

You are avoiding sprouts, cabbage, etc., but should eat what I am calling 'leafy greens'. Basically, if it is a leaf, it is OK. These include spinach, lettuce, lamb's lettuce, watercress and so on. You can also have chicory, peeled cucumber, courgettes and marrows. If in doubt, ask yourself if your vegetable came from under or above the ground. As this book sells all over the world, I am not being too prescriptive in case your diet includes some greens I have never heard of, but it is safe to eat all leaves. Do not include roots at this point. Root vegetables are higher carbohydrate and can cause a small but significant reaction in your system. By all means have them during the evening, but do not choose them for the daytime.

A standard portion of leafy greens has around 2g protein, a trace of fat and less than 1g carbohydrate.

Chicory has slightly higher carbohydrate, but that is per head of chicory.

Summary of Important Permitted Foods

**These foods can be eaten freely on your Maintenance programme,
but bear in mind the guidance on portion control**

Fish	Fowl	Meat	Dairy
salmon	skinned chicken	lamb	live 'bio' yoghurt
tuna	skinned turkey	pork	skimmed milk
smoked haddock**	pheasant	beef*	cottage cheese
smoked salmon**	duck	venison	hard cheese
white cod and haddock	goose	lean ham**	fromage frais
halibut	quail	lean bacon**	eggs
trout			
sardines			
prawns			
scallops			
crab			
lobster			

* Beef is digested slowly and can cause constipation.

** High in sodium and preservatives. Eat sparingly.

Vegetables – eat freely any time	lettuce, watercress, lamb's lettuce, peppers, rocket, radicchio, french or runner beans, courgette, avocado pear, chicory, spinach
Fruits – eat with care after 6 p.m.	grapes, apples, apricots, plums, stewed fruits, sieved, cooked fruits, blackcurrants, raspberries, mango, pineapple, strawberries, bananas, fruit mousses, all dried fruit
Fats and dressings – OK to eat in moderation	unsalted butter, half-fat crème fraiche, fresh mayonnaise, single or half-fat cream, olive oil, sunflower oil, walnut oil, sesame oil
Cereals – during the day eat these ones only	oats, Rice Krispies, Special K
Nuts – eat after 6 p.m. only	Brazil nuts, hazelnuts, almonds, unsalted cashew nuts, walnuts, sunflower seeds, pine nuts
Cereals – eat after 6 p.m. only, or avoid altogether	Shredded Wheat, Weetabix, rice, pasta, bran flakes, All-Bran
Vegetables – eat after 6 p.m. only	carrots, parsnip, swede, potatoes, tomatoes, sweetcorn, peas, broad beans

Exclude Completely

Vegetables	Fats – read labels or avoid	Miscellaneous
mushrooms	low-fat spreads – *do not eat*	*all* biscuits
baked beans	salted butter	cakes
butter beans	lard	muffins
kidney beans	bought mayonnaise	bagels
onions	with emulsifiers, etc.	baguettes
chickpeas		sweets
		bought mousses
		fruit yoghurts
		very low-fat or low-calorie yoghurts
		bought sandwiches
		'fast' food
		breadcrumbed products
		salted peanuts

Yeast-forming Foods

The following foods have a tendency to cause bloating. They are known as yeast-forming foods because they are held responsible for intestinal chaos that is sometimes a result of lingering bacterial infections, courses of antibiotics and taking the Pill or HRT treatment:

• peanuts

• pickles

• soy sauce

• tomato ketchup

• vinegar

• grapes and wine

• beer and lager

• dried fruits

• ice cream

• gravy mixes

• sweet potatoes

• mushrooms.

It is by no means inevitable that you are sensitive to these foods, but it will not hurt to leave them out altogether during your initial five days. There is plenty left to eat!

Cheese is included in the standard 5-Day programme, but do see how you get on with it as some people find it tricky. Cottage cheese is fine, but I suggest you steer clear of blue-veined cheeses.

Portion Control

Portion size is big news. Sizes have doubled and even quadrupled in the past twenty years. Burgers are three times the size they used to be. Even food outlets that have salad bars allow 'main meal' salads where you can pile your plate as high as you like and a whole generation is growing up with the notion that a twelve-inch (30cm) platter laden with an eight-ounce (225g) chicken breast, six roast potatoes, four tablespoons of each vegetable and a mound of stuffing is a standard meal.

I am afraid it is not. People constantly write to me in amazement at their weight gain and protruding stomach and tell me they are eating exactly the same as they ate ten years ago. They aren't.

They might be eating the same food, but they are almost certainly eating at least thirty per cent more of it.

If you are going to conquer your body, you need to conquer portions. The good news is that this is not going to mean a huge sacrifice. You will know by now that I hate substitute food and love the real thing. You might be shifting your meals around on the Grenfell programme but you are not sacrificing much. Rather than give up chicken in cream sauce, you will have a smaller portion. And with time, you will wonder how you ever managed to eat so much.

Here Are Your Portion Sizes:

Vegetables

- greens, carrots, etc. 2 tablespoons
- peas, broad beans 2 tablespoons
- mashed parsnips, carrots 2 tablespoons
- boiled or roast potatoes 2 small potatoes or 100g (3$\frac{1}{2}$oz)
- mashed potato with skimmed milk and a dot of butter 2 tablespoons or one scoop
- baked potato in its jacket 150g (5oz)

Pulses

- lentils 2 tablespoons

Salads

Your salad plate should be no bigger than 7 inches (18cm).
- salad greens 4–6 leaves
- cucumber 4 slices
- peppers 2–3 rings of each
- sweetcorn 1 tablespoon
- grated carrot 1 tablespoon
- radishes 1 tablespoon
- all other salad additions: keep portions small

Other

- chicken, beef steak, lamb or pork chop 150g (5oz)
- roasted meat 3 slices
- meat casserole 2 tablespoons
- pasta or rice 60g (2oz) dry weight
- bread 1 medium slice
- rice pudding and other puddings 3 tablespoons
  (should fit into a 120–150g/4–5oz yoghurt pot)
- stewed fruits 2–3 tablespoons
- fish standard fillet (about 125–180g/4–6oz)
- butter 60g (2oz) for the whole five days
- milk: as much as you need

the 5-DAY diet

This plan should be followed for five days.

It is important that you keep to the plan and do not try to find reasons why it will not work for you, for example not liking yoghurt or oats. This is like asking your doctor for different medication when he gives you the best cure for your problem. This diet is my best advice. If you decide to change it, I cannot guarantee the outcome.

The simplicity of the Grenfell programme not only helps you lose weight and reduce bloating, but it frees you from the stress of endless choices. However, if you want more variety, you can find suggestions for alternative meals on page 48.

Advance Preparation

Everybody is busy, so anything which you can prepare in advance helps you stay away from temptation in the kitchen.

Here are some suggestions:

1 Where possible, try to make or cook two or more of foods like poached salmon and grilled chicken breast, which are both nice to have cold in salads. You then have a portion ready for the next day. Batch-cooking is a sensible idea that has kept me going on my busy schedule for years.

2 Always have hard-boiled eggs and grated cheese handy in the fridge.

3 Weigh out your ration of butter and put it in a separate dish in the fridge ready for use. This is 60g (2oz) for five days, or 3oz (85g) for a week.

Tip

Puréed, mashed or stewed fruits and vegetables are a good shortcut to easing discomfort, bloating and wind. Sometimes you only need remove the peel or skin, but I have always found that well-puréed carrot, parsnip and even broccoli – as if you were making it for a baby – can reduce the wind factor. I discovered this years ago when making meals for my children. After the inevitable 'clearing up' of their leftovers, I didn't have any bloating! Some people yearn to have vegetables and fruit in their diet, but the tiniest spoonful blows them up, so either baby food or mashed/puréed fruit and vegetables are a good alternative. See if it works for you, because it is not guaranteed. *Experiment!*

Day 1

Breakfast Porridge, made with 30g (1oz) oats and water served with 1tsp honey, if desired, and skimmed milk
or
30g (1oz) porridge oats soaked in a teacup of skimmed milk, with 1 dsp plain yoghurt and a drizzle of honey

Mid-morning Small pot live natural yoghurt

Lunch 2 small slices chicken or beef
or
Half an avocado with prawns or a whole avocado
Mixed leaf salad with Vinaigrette (page 103) or oil-only dressing

Mid-afternoon Small pot live natural yoghurt
or
Milky coffee

Evening meal Poached or grilled fillet of salmon or cod (if salmon, cook one extra fillet and refrigerate)
Peas
Boiled potatoes or salad
or
Cheese Soufflé (page 100)

Dessert 6 prunes (tinned in fruit juice) or 8 sliced strawberries
Half-fat crème fraiche or fromage frais or Fresh Custard (page 104)

Supper
(if hungry) 1 apple
1 banana
6 almonds
(These can be whole or in a fruit salad)
Warm skimmed milk with honey

> Please do not forget that your water intake today and every day should be 2 litres (3½ pints). Drink water during the day at every opportunity.

Day 2

Breakfast	Porridge as on Day 1
	or
	2 poached eggs with 2 rashers bacon
Mid-morning	Glass of skimmed milk
	or
	Milky coffee
Lunch	Cold salmon (from yesterday)
	Mixed leaf salad
	Mayonnaise (page 103)
	or
	Cottage cheese and salad
Mid-afternoon	Small pot live natural yoghurt
Evening meal	Plain roast or grilled chicken breast
	(I suggest you cook two pieces of chicken and leave one to have cold for tomorrow)
	Boiled potatoes
	Broad bean salad
	Carrots
	or
	Cheese Omelette or Spinach Omelette made with 3 eggs (page 101)
	Jacket potato
	Sweetcorn
Dessert	6 large prunes
	or
	Mixed fruit salad of 1 banana, 12 grapes, $\frac{1}{2}$ apple
	Half-fat crème fraiche or fromage frais or Fresh Custard (page 104)
Supper (if hungry)	1 apple
	1 banana
	6 almonds
	(These can be whole or in a fruit salad)
	Warm skimmed milk and honey

Day 3

Breakfast

Porridge as on Day 1

or

30g (1oz) Rice Krispies, no sugar, 1 teacup skimmed milk

Mid-morning

Small pot live natural yoghurt

or

Milky coffee

Lunch

Cold chicken (from yesterday)

Green salad

Mayonnaise (page 103)

or

Herb Omelette Salad (page 101)

Mid-afternoon

Small mixed salad with Vinaigrette (page 103)

Evening meal

Salmon with Almond and Honey Crust (page 92) or Grilled salmon Florentine (on a bed of spinach)

Mashed potato

2 or 3 vegetables

or

Stir-fried mixed vegetables (courgette, peppers, carrots, etc)

4 tbsp cooked brown rice or mixed rice (Red Carmargue, Thai black rice, etc., as available)

Dessert

6 prunes with Rice Pudding (page 104)

or

3 pineapple slices, roasted, with half-fat crème fraiche or fromage frais or Fresh Custard (page 104)

Supper
(if hungry)

1 apple

1 banana

6 almonds

(These can be whole or in a fruit salad)

Warm skimmed milk and honey

Day 4

Breakfast
Porridge as on Day 1
or
30g (1oz) porridge oats soaked in a teacup of skimmed milk, with 1 dsp plain yoghurt and a drizzle of honey

Mid-morning
Small pot live natural yoghurt

Lunch
Caesar Salad (page 99)
or
Salade Niçoise (page 91)

Mid-afternoon
Half an avocado eaten from the shell

Evening meal
Cod in Parsley Sauce (page 91)
or
Roasted salmon fillet on a bed of spinach
Boiled potatoes
3 vegetables

Dessert
4 fresh pineapple slices with yoghurt
or
6 large prunes with half-fat crème fraiche or fromage frais or Fresh Custard (page 104)

Supper
(if hungry)
Stewed apple and blackberries with 1½ tbsp Fresh Custard (page 104)
or
1 apple
1 banana
6 almonds
(These can be whole or in a fruit salad)
Warm skimmed milk and honey

Day 5

Breakfast   Smoked salmon and scrambled eggs made with 3 eggs
or
Small pot live natural yoghurt with 1 tsp honey

Mid-morning   Very small leaf salad with shavings of Parmesan cheese and Vinaigrette
(page 103)

Lunch   Seafood platter – smoked salmon, prawns and crabmeat
Green salad with capers, etc.
Mayonnaise (page 103)
or
Smoked salmon and half an avocado with leaf salad
or
Cottage cheese with small sticks of carrot and celery
(this can cause wind – see how you feel)

Mid-afternoon   Small pot live natural yoghurt

Evening meal   Baked cod topped with tinned tomatoes
Mashed potato
Mashed parsnip (optional)
Peas
French beans or carrots
or
Cheese Omelette (page 101)
Sweetcorn and grated carrot
Boiled potatoes

Dessert   6 large prunes
or
Sliced fresh orange segments
Half-fat crème fraiche or fromage frais or Fresh Custard (page 104)

Supper
(if hungry)   1 apple
1 banana
6 almonds
(These can be whole or in a fruit salad)
Warm skimmed milk and honey

More Meal Choices

I have made your daily menus pretty rigid for the five days. Experience tells me that people prefer everything to be set down for them to follow. Sometimes, though, you need to be a little more flexible, so here are some other main meal ideas.

These are not to be eaten during the day. Keep them for after 6 p.m. when they can do less damage. I have not given recipes for all these meals as some will be familiar dishes you will be able to make without detailed instructions.

Chicken Roulade with Spinach (page 97) – on a mashed carrot and swede base

Grilled Chicken in Orange Marinade (page 95) – on mashed potato with peas

Chicken with a Pine Nut Crust (page 96) – on a bed of mashed, lightly buttered parsnips with a side mixed-leaf salad with Vinaigrette (page 103)

Warm Chicken and Potato Salad (page 107)

Chicken Malibu Salad (page 98)

Coconut Chicken Curry (page 96) – on a bed of grated carrot or green salad leaves with steamed jasmine rice

Spicy, Yoghurt-Baked Chicken (page 97)

Coronation Chicken (page 98)

Spinach Soufflé (page 100) – with a crisp salad and boiled potatoes

Ham and cheese omelette - with a mixed pepper salad

Spinach and ham omelette – with dry-roast potatoes

Barbecued Salmon with Citrus (page 93) – with a crisp salad

Smoked Haddock and Smoked Salmon Fishcakes with Dill Cream (page 94) – with salad and peas

Sesame or Pine Nut Salmon with Orange (page 93) – with mashed spinach

Cod Florentine (page 90) – with carrots and cauliflower

Baked Cheese Tomatoes (page 101) – with a jacket potato

Exercise and Posture

Doing It the Natural Way

If you want to succeed with your fabulously flat stomach, you have to get moving. These days 'exercise' has come to mean something rather formal at the gym, but the difference between exercise and movement is like the difference between taking your dog for a walk on a lead, and simply opening the door to let it wander round the garden. Both would have the same result. In the same way, all types of movement count as exercise and if you are relying on daily sit-ups to flatten that tummy for you, you might have to wait rather a long time.

Put it like this: there are twenty-four hours in a day and if you only tone your abs for fifteen minutes a day, that leaves a lot of time for them to get out of shape! The great thing about natural movement is (a) you don't realize you are doing it, (b) it's instant and free, (c) it gets better results because your muscles are being toned all the time. The Grenfell 5-Day programme puts great store by natural effort, a healthy lifestyle and the great outdoors. You can walk anywhere at any time. Go out to post a letter, rather than saving it for when you drive by the box. Cancel the newspaper delivery and walk or jog to the shop instead. If you are concerned about safety, go mall-walking: that's walking round your local shopping centre where you have stairs, a climate-controlled environment and loos!

I am very much an outdoors person and urge you to try it for yourself. It is so great for your figure and you get several jobs done at once – gardening or shopping or whatever plus a wonderful flat stomach.

Completing the Circle

Working on your abs to the exclusion of everything else will only do a third of the job. The whole abdominal section of your body is what I call your 'midcircle' and you must exercise the whole of it. You will target:

- your oblique muscles (the ones that run down the side of your trunk)

- your rectus abdominis muscle (the one that if overdeveloped forms the 'six-pack' appearance)

- your hip flexors (they start at your hips and run down your legs and can help to tone your lower abdominal area)

- your back muscles – to help you stand up straight without thinking about it.

In order of effectiveness, here are my top exercises for the midcircle:

1 Swimming
This tones all your muscles, moves joints in their full range, stretches and tones your abdominals and obliques and strengthens your back.

2 Sweeping, raking, hoovering
Really hard sweeping or raking is good for your abdominals as long as you remember to pull in your tummy before you start. Thereafter, each sweeping move towards you contracts your abdominals.

3 Washing the floor
I don't know if you have ever seen or used an ab-roller, but washing a floor on hands and knees is the same movement that you would get using one of those toning gadgets. You need to be on your knees, reaching out with one arm and then the other, or both together. The act of reaching and then drawing your arms towards you on the floor is fabulous for toning your abs. Five minutes is enough.

Which Exercise?

It is always assumed that if people simply take more exercise their figure problems will disappear. If only. Cycling will not improve your abdominals, neither will step aerobics. You need the right exercise for your own needs and, right now, we want a flatter stomach.

If you are a complete beginner, if you have health problems, bad knees and have never walked further than the kitchen, you won't want to wade straight in with 100 sit-ups before breakfast. But neither will you welcome my suggestion of a gentle morning stroll if you've just completed the London Marathon. The main thing to do, though, is to increase whatever you are doing now, and to do more floor exercises every day. So if you are doing nothing in the way of exercise, it's best to start with about five minutes of warm-up and stomach-tightening exercises, adding some aerobic exercise every day. If you are a hot-shot expert, go the whole hog with advanced abdominal exercises five times a day, and an extra forty-five minutes of aerobic work such as swimming or cycling. Whatever you are doing, do more of it!

Muscle Toning – What Is It?

Every muscle is toned simply by being moved. Toning just means it is doing something. People will often 'tone' themselves with weights, but weights build muscle, adding to their size and capability. When you do your midcircle exercises, I want you to tone your muscles, not build them. Building them will result in bigger muscles and you could even find your waist thickening and your abdomen bulging.

This is not as fanciful as it sounds. A friend of mine went from flab to fab eight years ago, but got hooked on her ever flatter tummy. Soon she was adding weights to her sit-up routines and doing those exercises where you hang by your knees from a bar and sit up – holding twenty-pound (9kg) weights! Needless to say, she had an impressive six-pack. Sadly, these days she is nearly fifty and her workouts are naturally less energetic, but that six-pack has turned into a fat-free but loose set of muscles, hanging limp as a spare tyre under her T-shirt. Not a good look. On this plan, you will be toning your muscles with your own bodyweight.

GrenFlex

You can't look good if you don't stretch. Modern ways of exercising have left women with bowed, muscular thighs, thick ankles and large calves. Many women would call themselves fit, yet they can't straighten their knees. Nor can they press a hand into the space between their shoulder blades or touch their toes. They might have a body–fat ratio to die for, but total fitness includes having muscles that can operate over a large range and that means they should be flexible and easily stretched to avoid injury. An individual who is fit but not flexible cannot be said to have all-round fitness.

Beauty is an entire effect. Some people train themselves into the ground for the body beautiful, then shower and slouch off with their sports bag weighing down their shoulders. No thought of elegance. No line to the body or beauty of movement. No point.

Flexibility training should be included as part of your daily activities from now on and that is why I have introduced GrenFlex bands. They are a specific resistance and length and are your ultimate tool for stretching, lengthening and toning that midcircle – and all in one tiny band that you can pack in your luggage when you travel. A flat stomach depends on having a nice line to your body with long, lean and stretched muscles. With GrenFlex you lengthen your abdominals and waist and can improve the appearance of your stomach by several inches.

Now, you do not have to use a GrenFlex band. If you are elderly, not physically strong because you have been ill or simply do not wish to have a band, you don't have to use one. Your normal abdominal exercises from the next section will be quite enough to flatten your abs and give you noticeably toned muscles.

However, there is no substitute for the band, as it is immensely strong and will not snap, allowing extremes of safe movement.

A Quick Calorie Count

I don't approve of counting calories for the sake of it, but just for fun, and to cheer you up if you are stuck in an office or at home and can't get out much, here is a list of the calories spent doing a variety of ordinary chores:

Calories per half-hour:

Sleeping 30

Sweeping 90

Making beds 120

Typing 60

Standing still 45

Driving 60

Eating 45

Mowing the lawn 225

Washing dishes 60

Digging the garden 240

Washing clothes 90

Moderate cycling 120

Writing 60

Racing cycling 330

Ironing 60

Squash 420

Knitting 45

Aerobics 200–300

Mopping the floor 120

Brisk walking 180

Exercising at Home

I admit that I am probably the vainest woman in England! I was conscious of wanting a good figure even when my children were small. With limited time and absolutely no facilities or babysitters, I did what everybody did – got down on the floor for five precious minutes when the children were napping and did my stretch and sit-up routine.

The Grenfell 5-Day programme was born from those days. This is a plan that works because it is about consistency rather than an unsustainable effort every six months. Think of it like a fantastic hairdo. If you had a killer cut and expensive restyle would you expect it to look just as good after three months? Of course not. Would you blame the hairdresser and say the hairstyle 'didn't work' if it was a total mess after a few weeks? You'd be mad to. But people say this all the time about diet and exercise plans which they have tried for a couple of months and then given up on. They say it didn't work.

Don't save all your exercise for the gym. Exercising at home is sensible body-maintenance which you have to do.

Here is your exercise programme:

Always warm up

The purpose of a warm-up is to prepare the body for exercise. Muscles which are cold – and remember that even on the hottest day your muscles will not be ready for action if they have been at rest – will not stretch, and will tear easily.

Your Five Abdominal Exercises

I am going to give you just five variations on the standard stomach-strengthening exercise. They are:

1 the Foundation

2 the Crunch

3 the Waist Whittler

4 the Chair Lift

5 the Air Bike.

You do not have to do all the variations.
If you are new to abdominal exercise, if you have been ill or have had a baby, it is best to stay with the Foundation exercise until you are stronger. It will be quite enough to keep you toned and trim, and as you progress you can add in the Waist Whittler, which is another quite basic exercise. If you are already accustomed to exercise, I suggest you do all five exercises twice a day on alternate days.

Abdominal exercises are not always easy to get right. People complain that their neck aches and their back hurts. If anything ever hurts, stop at once. There can be several reasons for the pain:

1 Your position is wrong.

2 You have done too many repetitions.

3 You are tired.

4 It is the wrong time of the month.

This last reason is important because your monthly cycle can affect the way you exercise to quite a marked degree. In the week or so before your period, hormones are pouring into your body that mimic pregnancy in a small way, and your ligaments can be a little vulnerable. Around this time, women can suffer from minor injuries more easily than at other times, so take care.

The Foundation

1 Start off lying down with your feet flat on the floor, about hip-width apart.
2 Place both hands under the bulge at the back of your head. Look at the ceiling.
3 Lift your head, but let your hands take its weight.
4 Make your chest and your head and neck one piece, in one line. The best way to think of your upper position is that the line of your top half should not be broken by the hinge of the neck.
5 Inhale before you start. Exhale, as you press your stomach downwards towards the floor. Tilt your pelvis up towards your chest and neck. Lift your head without breaking the line by tugging on your head or jerking it upwards. Keep pressing your stomach down.

   This pattern of breathing should continue throughout. Breathe in before you start, or on the release of effort. Breathe out and press downwards at the point of maximum effort, i.e. when you lift. Breathe in as you slowly and gently lower your head back down towards the floor.

6 Good! Now you have mastered the form of the sit-up, do eight more repetitions.
7 Have a rest for ten seconds; bring your knees into your chest.
8 Repeat the exercise, doing eight or sixteen repetitions, according to how you feel.
9 Stretch out by turning over and lifting yourself on to your elbows. Remember to keep your head and neck in alignment with your spine by looking down at the floor while you do this.

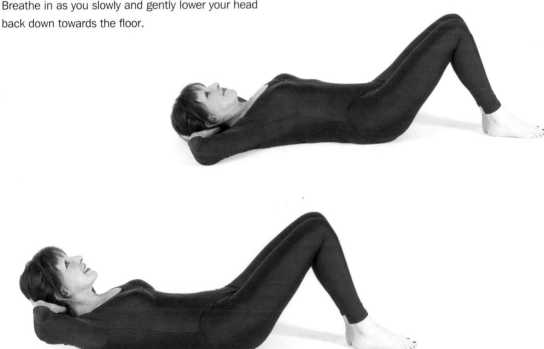

The Crunch

1 This time, lie on the floor with your feet lifted off the floor and cross your ankles. Feel the small of your back pressed firmly to the floor.
2 Take your upper position, as for the Foundation, neck and chest in one line. Support your head with your hands. As before, do not pull on your neck. Your head and back should be in one line.
3 Breathe in, lift your chest and press your stomach downwards, exhaling as you do so. Lift and lower your head as in the Foundation four times, up and down, slowly, then do eight double-time pulses, then repeat the four slow crunches.
4 Turn over and stretch out as before to decompress your spine.

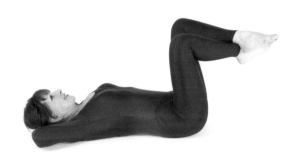

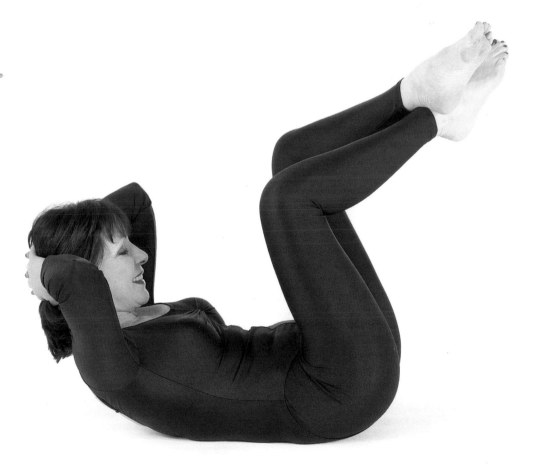

The Chair Lift

This exercise is slightly easier than the Crunch if you find it hard to keep your legs up. It also stops your legs from helping you, thereby giving your stomach muscles all the hard work!

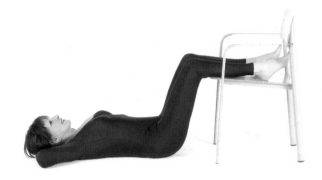

1 Lie on the floor with your bottom about 45cm (18 inches) from the base of a chair. Place your legs from the knee downwards on the chair. Put your hands under your head as in the previous exercises.
2 Breathe in to prepare. Breathe out, and press downwards with your abdomen, raising your upper body as you do so. You won't come up very high.
3 Lower as you breathe in, expanding your chest as you do so. Repeat eight times, rest and repeat a further eight.
4 Turn over and decompress your spine as before.
5 Return to your starting position and repeat the two sets of eight. Decompress.

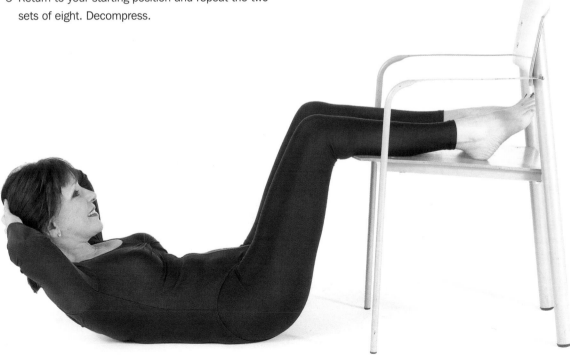

The Air Bike

Only do this exercise if you are not severely overweight, and if you can be sure to keep your legs up in the air. It isn't a failing if you find it hard – you'll work up to it soon enough!

1 Take position as in picture.
2 Pulse slowly up to each knee with the opposite elbow as it comes in towards your face, then stretch the leg out towards the ceiling. Do eight or sixteen slowly, depending on your level of fitness and strength.
3 Rest, repeat the set then turn over to stretch out, decompressing as before.

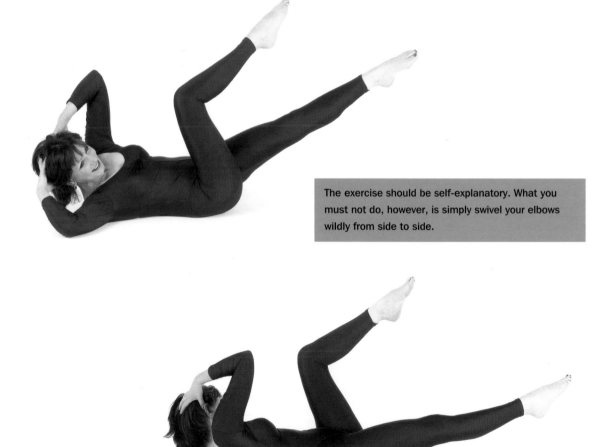

The exercise should be self-explanatory. What you must not do, however, is simply swivel your elbows wildly from side to side.

The Waist Whittler

Without exercise, your oblique muscles, which lie around your ribcage area and which shape your waist, sit there, do nothing and are slack. This exercise does not increase the number of muscle fibres because you are not using weight. It tones and stretches the muscles so they become taut, and give you a tighter, smaller waist.

1 Lie on your back, arms outstretched. Lift your feet off the floor, as shown, knees bent. Press your spine hard to the floor and breathe in.
2 Now breathe out as you allow your legs to roll to one side, slowly. Keep your legs touching all the time. Stop short of the floor or go as far as you can. Hold and breathe in again, tightening your abdominal muscles and checking the position of your shoulders, which should still be on the floor.
3 Breathe out and, using your torso muscles, bring your legs back to centre and then over to the opposite side. Repeat this move slowly, about three times to each side. If you can do more, great. But you must keep both shoulders on the floor so that your waist and hips have to do the work!
4 Turn over and decompress your spine as before.

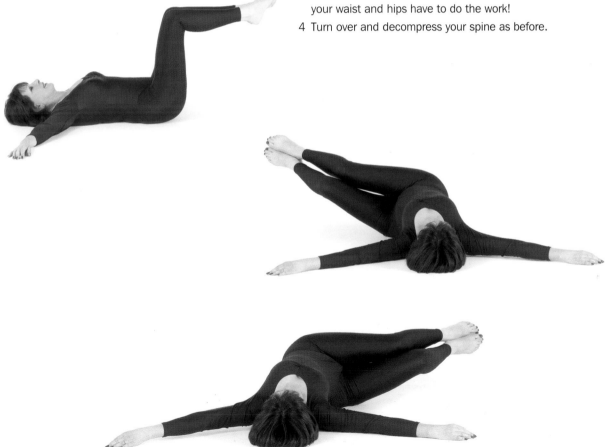

GrenFlex Flexibility Exercises with a Band

Most people I have given a band to end up almost addicted to it! What I love about the bands is that absolutely anybody can do some sort of exercise with them and you can certainly master exercises which would be inconceivable without them. For example, working the lower abs. A movement you will see in a minute, with legs outstretched and arms over your head, would be almost impossible without a band for anyone but the super-fit. It could hurt your back. But with a band you are supported while being stretched and you can adapt the move as you get stronger so your abs really are taking most of the strain. Then you get results! For now, I just want you to get to love the band as much as I do. You can buy a band from my website, www.monicagrenfell.co.uk.

For now, let's see how you hold it.

Any exercise with the band is made slightly harder by shortening your band, increasing resistance. You can either wind it round your hands a couple more times or bring your hands closer together.

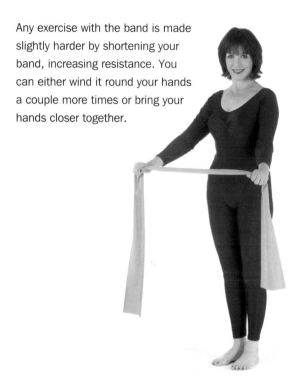

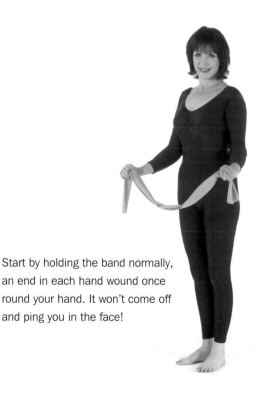

Start by holding the band normally, an end in each hand wound once round your hand. It won't come off and ping you in the face!

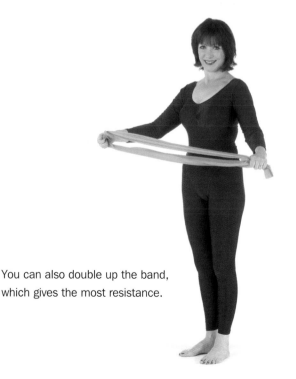

You can also double up the band, which gives the most resistance.

Now stand straight, or you can sit on a stool without arms or on the floor.

Fold the band double.

Raise your arms above your head, pulling gently outwards on the band as you do so.

Allow your arms to go backwards as far as you can and if you are able, drop your arms behind your back. Stand or sit up straight and feel the stretch in your shoulders. This is lifting your ribcage, stomach muscles and waist.

Come back to the centre and lean slightly to one side. Keep stretching your arms apart. If you are sitting, keep both buttocks on the floor or stool. Hold and breathe. Breathe in and then out as you take your arms up and over to the other side. Breathe evenly.

You can also sit on the centre of the band, using its full length. Pick up the left hand side with your right hand and bring the band up the side of your body. You should feel a great stretch in the right side of your waist as the band tries to pull you over to your left. Hold, and then repeat on the other side.

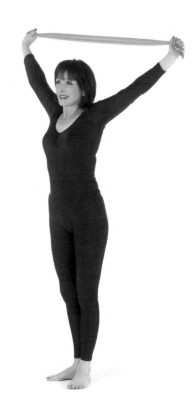

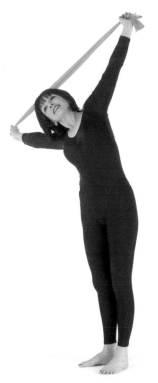

Exercise 1

Lie with your back flat on the floor with your knees in to your chest and the band under the soles of your feet. You might want to wear soft rubber-soled shoes for this – I use bare feet or soft jazz shoes, but you will get less flexibility if you wear trainers. The band should not slip, and even if it does it won't hurt you.

1 Hold arms in a bicep-curl position.
2 Now stretch out your legs at an angle keeping arms still. Keep your back pressed down to the floor. Bring knees in again and repeat six times. Relax for twenty seconds.
3 Repeat six times.

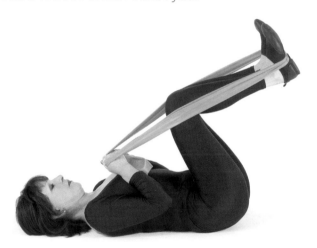

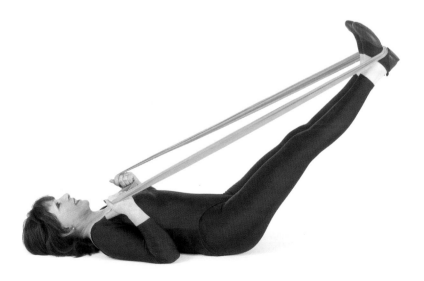

Exercise 2

1 From the same starting position, this time raise your arms above your head. Do six. Relax for twenty seconds.
2 Repeat six times.

Repeat exercises 1 and 2 again.

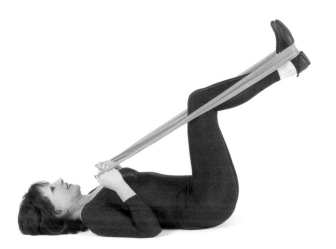

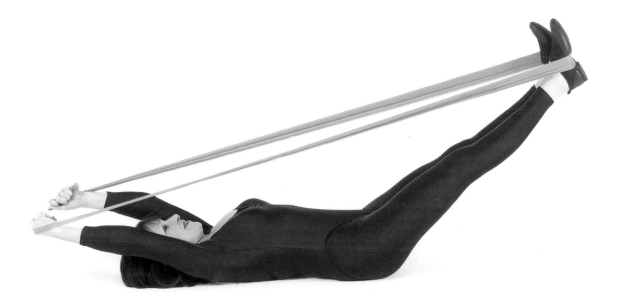

Exercise 3

1 From the same starting position, raise your arms high and lift your shoulders off the floor. Hold. Release and repeat six times. Relax for twenty seconds.
2 Repeat.

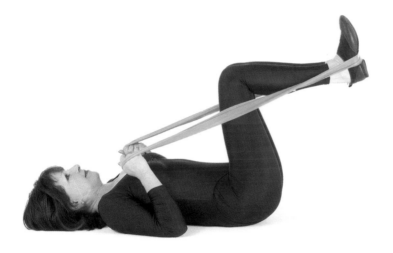

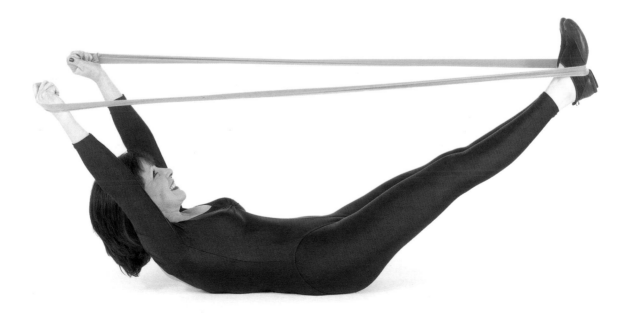

Exercise 4

1 Place the band under your right foot and hold
   the ends in your right hand. Stretch the leg up to
   the ceiling to start; getting a nice hamstring stretch
   while you are there!
2 Slowly lengthen your leg and reach arm overhead.
   This stretches your entire side torso and gives you
   an extra good stretch for your lower abdominal and
   hip flexor areas.

Do six times, change legs and repeat. Hold each
stretch for twenty seconds, trying to extend the stretch
all the time.

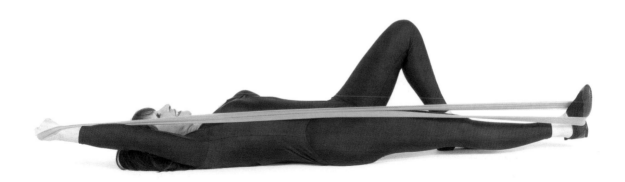

Exercise 5

1 Turn over onto your front. Double the band and hold as I am doing. Breathe in.
2 Breathe out as you lift your head and shoulders from the floor, extending and pulling the band wide as you do so. You won't go far.
3 Hold for a few seconds, then relax back to the floor. Try to lift and hold even further each time.

This exercise is wonderful for posture and will strengthen and tone your back muscles.

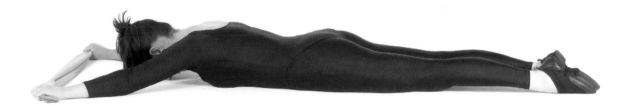

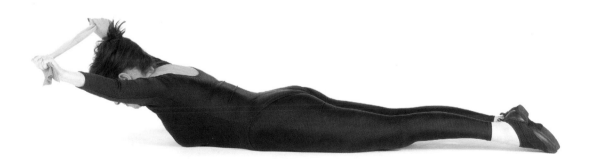

Frequency of Exercise

Never work the same muscles two days running.
What I suggest you do, not just for your first five days but
for the future, is a weekly programme along these lines:

Day 1 Full programme of toning and GrenFlex exercises,
plus 45-minute run or walk.

Day 2 30-minute swim.

Day 3 Aerobics video such as my *Get Back into Your Jeans*
50-minute workout. (Can be ordered on my website.)

Day 4 Full programme of abdominal and GrenFlex exercises.

Day 5 45-minute run or walk.

Days 6 and 7 Rest, but keep moving. Gentle walking,
sports or household jobs.

Your Posture Is Terrible!

There is no point in losing weight if you are going to ruin the effect by slouching. Exercising your body to perfection, dieting yourself into the ground and spending a fortune on clothes are time and money wasted if your chest droops, your neck caves in and your stomach sticks out – all because you don't stand properly.

Good posture is most noticeable when you don't have it. Not only is it important for your look – bad posture suggests depression, lack of confidence, boredom – but it affects your digestion, breathing and general health. Bad posture places strain on ligaments and muscles leading to pain, stiffness, and general lack of mobility.

Nearly everything we do pulls our bodies inwards and downwards, contributing to poor posture. We are designed to face one way and all our movements lead in that direction – inwards and downwards. We bend down, lean forwards. We have no occasion to lean backwards, or to carry out a task with our hands behind our backs. We were meant to live on all fours.

I was standing at the supermarket checkout the other day behind a woman who had a trim bottom encased in skintight jeans, a snug T-shirt and who held great promise of being just as gorgeous from the front. When she finally turned round, my jaw nearly dropped open because she had a particularly prominent stomach. This was not just your average little bulge, and she clearly was not pregnant. Her chest slouched down to her navel, her bust hung unattractively and her stomach protruded. And this was all down to posture.

Good posture is a habit. One of the worst things you can do is to stand for a long time. The natural tendency when standing is to lean backwards, but this conjures up pictures of slanting bodies that look as if they are compensating for a stiff breeze. What we do is stick our hips forwards and balance the top half of our body on top of our pelvis, so the socket joints of our hips are taking all the strain of the pelvis. Do it and you will see what I mean. This pushes your stomach forwards and there you have your sticking-out stomach. It takes a conscious effort to pull yourself back into alignment, but conscious effort is what the Grenfell 5-Day programme is all about. Below you can see the typical backwards lean of the body at rest. It causes what is known as 'kyphosis'.

Kyphosis

Rounded shoulders are often the result of tight chest muscles, which can be the result of slumping over a desk all day or of overdeveloping them with a gym routine. Many women work their pectoral muscles into the ground in the expectation of getting perkier boobs, but this pulls the shoulders forwards and can cause a hunched back. Look at bodybuilders' shoulders and back, which tend to be extremely rounded.

Note the effect on the abdomen.

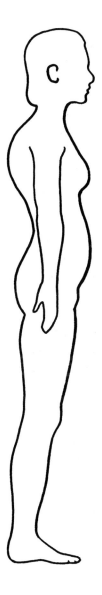

The Dowager's Hump

This postural fault is caused by a poor sitting position over a period of time, common in office workers and schoolchildren. The chin juts forward and the upper spine curves to compensate. The abdominal muscles are unable to work properly and the pelvis tips backwards, resulting in a sagging appearance. Note that the figure shown is not overweight, yet the stomach appears large and unsightly.

Apart from your hairstyle and weight, nothing is more ageing than poor posture. Rightly or wrongly, we associate stooped figures with old people, and next time you see someone who seems young for their age, make a note of what it is about them that gives this impression. It is not just good skin, hair or slimness. A sprightly step and a good carriage are what mark people out as looking younger. A sagging stomach suggests neglect, fatigue and a generally lacklustre attitude to life. We have all seen women in their twenties looking like this. Standing properly lifts your ribcage and flattens your stomach.

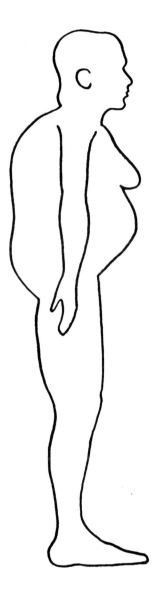

Get into the habit of practising your posture in front of a full-length mirror every morning. It will soon become second nature.

Do these posture reminders every day.

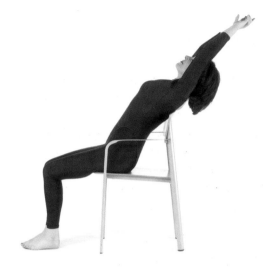

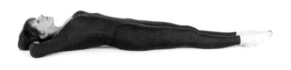

1 Lie on your back. Place your hands behind your head and press the elbows down to touch the floor.

2 Sit in a chair as shown and have a nice stretch backwards. This decompresses your spine from its usual bent-forwards position.

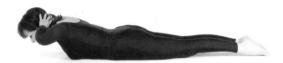

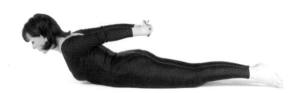

Alternatively, lying on your stomach you can clasp your hands behind your head as shown and stretch upwards and back. If you have tight shoulders this is slightly easier.

Where Do I Go from Here?

The Grenfell Lifetime Maintenance Programme

After your 5-Day plan, you are probably feeling great and you want to keep that feeling going. With the Grenfell Maintenance Programme, you can. But it's time for a bit of reality. If this has been a simple programme to help you lose those vanity pounds (the ones only you know are there!) that's fine. If you just wanted to banish bloating, I hope you have learned a few tricks. If ever you feel bloated, think about what you have been eating and try to identify your particular culprits and avoid including these in your own cooking. If, however, you need to lose weight and this is a big undertaking, you need to look at a few other aspects of your life.

And the great news is that you don't have to eat yoghurt forever or save fruit until the evening. If you have a special date, fine: you know what to do. My Maintenance programme, on the other hand, allows a sensible, controlled diet so you can still lose weight at the same time as keeping your bottom line daily in view on a daily basis. A too-strict diet would be hard to manage, but the Maintenance programme allows a little leeway within your five steps.

The 5-point Lifetime Maintenance Plan

Having been on the receiving end of thousands of letters
and emails from my readers over the years, and having been
a private diet counsellor to many women, I have often heard
the phrase 'Where am I going wrong?' It usually comes after
yet another diet has failed, although as I said at the beginning
of this book, diets can't fail. It is like saying a car is fast – it
all depends on who drives it.

Where people go wrong is in not having a proper plan. A diet
sheet with a list of meals isn't going to get you through the next
crisis or relationship break-up. A few breakfast ideas won't
motivate you back onto your diet after a binge. Your problem
is still there. So I have devised a 5-point plan that goes beyond
the diet to provide a lifetime programme to deal with your
weight problems.

1 Start again – get rid of the past.

2 Define your bottom line – who do you want to be?

3 Set your midline – what you are going to do to achieve it?

4 Tell somebody that you want to change. Ask for their support.

5 Congratulate yourself – every day.
   Give thanks that you have learned to respect your body,
   what you eat and how you treat yourself.

1 Starting Again

I already talked about getting rid of the past: treating your house like you just moved in and the old you moved out. You want to chuck out all her old rubbish and get your new stuff in. You have to do this in your head, too.

Forget wallowing in childhood problems, dreadful parents or school bullying. They were ghastly and awful but you can't do anything about them now. Don't let them mess up the future. The past was once the future and you did not know what was coming. The future will soon be the past, so don't make it something you look back on and wish it could have been different. Change your past now by changing your future.

Say your farewells to the old you. It sounds corny, but some people find it helps to write a letter to themselves saying goodbye. Imagine you are saying this to a friend who is going a long way. Or maybe a relationship you want to finish and this is your letter to call it a day. Go on, write to yourself. You can even post it! If you prefer, post it to me at PO Box 64, Oxon OX12 9GA. It will be in complete confidence and you can be anonymous, but at least you will have told somebody.

If this sounds like the worst kind of psychobabble, believe me – I am the last person to indulge in that sort of thing. I am a practical, down-to-earth sort of woman. But having seen the effect this 'farewell' can have on clients of mine, I am happy to recommend it. Who cares what it is called as long as it works for you?

2 Find Your Bottom Line

You know the term the 'bottom line'? If you aren't familiar with it, it means the final analysis – what something is really about. So what is your life really about? What do you want, what do you want to achieve or be like? What is your bottom line?

It could be something simple, like 'I want to be a size ten' or 'I want to be healthier.' It could be more defined, like 'I want a 26-inch waist' or 'I don't want to be the fat mother of the bride.'

Defining your bottom line is a key stage on your programme. It is the reason you are doing it – to change your ways and become a person you are happier with. When things go haywire in the future, let a friend in on the secret and have them ask you, 'What's your bottom line?' Repeating it to yourself when you feel low will actually help you get back on track. Write it here:

I . . .

It might seem silly to write here in the book like a schoolgirl, but nobody will see it. And I cannot tell you how useful it will become in the future! Psychologists say that people who stop short of their full weight loss do so because they forget how they felt at the start. It is easy to feel satisfied with less, because the frustration, the anger, the disappointment in yourself, have faded. At any time, you can look back at this page, and seeing your writing will remind you how you felt when you wrote it. It is just a gentle reminder of your ambition for yourself.

a) What do you have to do?

Losing excess fat is the best thing you can do for your body. Getting a body you love is the pathway to success. Having a permanent, lifestyle diet is common sense. After all, you get a hairstyle which suits you best, a fashion sense and, with any luck, a partner who seems a good bet. Why not settle for a personal diet style that keeps you slim without your having to think about it?

A midline is what you have to do – the bare minimum that you are prepared to stick to for the rest of your life – new habits if you will. Basically, there is a set of rules that you are already familiar with which are the basis for success. These include:

- eat regularly

- eat slowly

- chew all food to a paste before swallowing

- eat smaller meals

- eat only at a table

- eat a good fruit supper

- drink a glass of water after every visit to the loo

- don't eat when stressed or argumentative

- practise good posture daily

- exercise in some way for at least 45 minutes five times a week

- do abdominal exercises three times a week.

b) Dropping below the line

Dropping below your midline can also be described as 'cheating' or 'falling off the wagon' or maybe just 'forgetting yourself'. It might not be major. But if you are intending to devote your life to looking good you have to know and admit when you have let yourself down. I do not want to sound fixated and obsessed at this point, but if you applied this principle to your work it would make sense. Skimping on a report, sneaking home early, sliding in late – it's all a bit below-the-midline of what is expected of you. It happens all the time with my clients and it usually results in overeating and weight gain. Try these reasons for dropping below the line:

- I was away from home on a business trip – nothing was normal.

- I was stressed.

- Someone died.

- My pet was ill.

- My children were playing up.

- It was my time of the month.

- I'm on the change and it's hell.

- I'm unhappy at work.

- My relationship's a mess.

Now this is difficult. All those circumstances are triggers. They are genuine triggers. But if you wait for everything to go right you might as well wait for ever, because it isn't going to happen. You and I know that hardly a week goes by when everything is perfect. So you need to get systems in place for eating and managing your diet so your relationship with food carries on as usual when everything around you is chaos. But you can still build in some flexibility. Your limitations can be something like this:

- On business trips, I will have whatever is available on the menu, but no desserts. Although chips and bread are below the line, it's OK if I have one or the other, but not both.

- When it's my time of the month and I give in to cravings, I will just have raw vegetables – they are not supposed to be on my programme, but they are better than ice cream or crisps!

- When I am a guest I will eat what I am given and if it is full-fat milk or sugary cereal, I won't make a fuss, go hungry or eat less when I get home.

- I can have three drinks a day on special occasions, but no more.

Add your own below-the-line get-out clauses, but recognize that they are the exception, not the rule!

c) Going above the line

Going one better than your rules is a short step to diet mania. It is easily done. You eat less one day, your weight dips and you are thrilled. You think that by eating even less you can speed that weight loss on its way. *Don't!*

This is not above the line or even good. If you have an encouraging weight loss one week, you will have another one the next week. Do not reward yourself by withholding food; do a bit extra for yourself instead, like:

- trying out a new healthy gourmet recipe

- buying something new to wear

- dressing stylishly to enhance your new figure

- practising walking and sitting elegantly to show your body and clothes to advantage

- buying better food instead of microwave meals.

Write down a few ideas. For example, you might once have thought shellfish and melon was a silly little meal that could not fill anyone up, but now you fancy something a little better than a jacket potato. Readers often tell me that they had never fancied avocado or could not imagine being satisfied with a spot of soufflé, but now they are hooked. Be prepared to amaze yourself and cook up something special.

d) Falling out of line

I hope you don't find yourself in this place. Overeating happens to all of us, but distinguishing between what is acceptable and what is not is a vital lesson.

Food is precious. Whatever your shortcomings, unhappiness or stresses, many people have nothing to eat and we are lucky to have plenty. Overeating by finishing off a cake or tub of ice cream is one thing: bingeing is another. Bingeing is never acceptable and you should not hand over responsibility for this bad habit by blaming circumstances. *You know what is right and what is wrong.*

Overeating immobilizes you. You become locked in your own world where you think about nothing but food and nobody but yourself. Eating to escape loneliness, anxiety, sadness or dissatisfaction with your life are characterized by:

- letting your self-image slip

- telling lies about what you have eaten

- looking for escapes

- blowing up at people

- making excuses for yourself

- blaming others for your lapses.

What you must do

1 Phone someone and talk about something else. Get out of yourself.

2 Look at your bottom line statement and remind yourself how you felt when you wrote it.

3 Forget what you ate. Wallowing in self-pity is wrong.

4 Match every excuse to a solution – it's OK to have reasons for bad things, but make sure you have a positive solution to end on. For example, 'I got stuck in traffic and was too late to exercise' translates to, 'I'll leave earlier tomorrow.'

5 Get back on your midline tomorrow and do not look back.

Everyone falls out of line sometimes. However, it is not a good place to be and you do not want to go there if you can avoid it. *You can avoid it.*

4 Tell Somebody

Tell somebody that you have decided to change. It is no different from deciding to give up being a business-woman in order to become a nurse.

You have every right to a makeover, so tell somebody that you are taking yourself in hand and would appreciate his or her support. Make them realize that this is serious. You have not been happy for some time with the way you eat, your lack of discipline, your health and fitness. Tell somebody that you are trying a new way but you don't want to make a big thing about it. If they are a good friend, they will understand.

The final part of this step is, *Don't go on about it*. This is not a slimming club where you band together and chat about how much chocolate you managed not to eat. Keep it to yourself and get on with it.

5 Congratulate Yourself

The Flatter Stomach programme is not easy. You will often see friends out having a good time, knocking back drinks and enjoying a takeaway. You can't do this. So how do you cope when things seem unfair and how can you congratulate yourself for your self-denial?

Well, for a start, you certainly aren't denying yourself anything except bad health, bad breath and a hangover. Anyway, you have been denying yourself a lot of good things for a long time: nice clothes, smaller sizes, compliments, confidence, self-esteem . . . it's a long list. Denying yourself a cake or some chocolate or a few vodka tonics, on the other hand, is a feeling that lasts a few minutes. Congratulate yourself that you have seen the difference!

Then there is the tricky question of those lucky friends who can eat and drink to their heart's content and get away with it. They break all the diet rules, live on junk and look a million dollars. Well, I have met these people too and they rarely look good for long. Anyway, we all have different talents and this is how you must see it. Some people sail through exams while others struggle. Some girls have fantastic hair without trying while others need every conditioner on the market. You can grow your nails long and some people never manage. So what?

Stop thinking about what other people do – this is about YOU.

Think about who you are. You want a flat stomach, you want a slim body and you want to lose weight or keep the figure you have. These are all admirable ambitions because they mean you are taking care of yourself and have pride in your appearance. Losing excess weight is the best thing you can do for your body. Feeling slim and confident will open doors. Congratulate yourself that you are willing to work at it.

Keep Up the Good Work

Keep Exercising!

You have only done five days of this diet so far, but you will have already found that not only does it work, that your stomach is feeling much, much flatter, but that you need less food on your plate. If you want to continue the diet for a further five days, go back to Day 1 and repeat the diet faithfully, or substitute a new evening meal or lunch each day from the recipe section. *All* the meals in this book are suitable for your diet; it is the size of *portion* that matters most in weight loss.

Try also to make or buy the best food you can afford. It need not cost a lot. Do insist on only eating pure, 'honest' food without a lot of chemicals added. Get a few great habits, like making your own bread. I make all my own simply because I will not allow manufacturers to push all those chemicals and bloating additives down my throat. It is not a chore because I make a huge quantity and freeze it, so I only bake once every few months. My unbleached white bread is famous round here, and I have given you a good recipe for it.

Your figure is important to you. That flat stomach feels wonderful. If you give up now, you'll be holding in your stomach for the rest of your life, choosing seats where your stomach is best hidden, wearing clothes you hate. You don't want to feel like that. For the sake of a little self-discipline you can have the body of your dreams, *every day*!

No diet can exercise your muscles. Fat loss won't mobilize your joints. See exercise for its own sake, not as some calorie-burning procedure. The calories you eat are for your health and growth and the calories you burn are for your cardio health.

If it is dark and cold and raining outside you might be tempted to stay in by the fire. *Don't!* The fire is all the better to come back to if you have been out at a fitness class or having a game of badminton or even a walk to the postbox. Losing weight is fine, but your figure matters too! You don't want to get to summer and find that you're ashamed of your stomach because it's still flabby, despite having lost all that weight.

Eating Out

When You Are a Guest

1 Never say you're on a diet, as it just goads people into making a comment.

2 Never say 'only a little, please' or 'just a small portion for me', as it alerts people to the fact that you're being careful. Take whatever you are given, eat your usual smaller portion and enjoy it.

3 Never worry about leaving food. You don't owe anybody an explanation of why you are not eating something, and if you are asked if the meal was all right, smile very brightly and say 'Yes thank you, it was delicious!'

4 Try not to have second helpings, except if etiquette demands that you keep another diner company.

5 Don't refuse anything unless you genuinely don't like it. Once everyone is into the swing of the evening they won't have a clue whether you've eaten it or not.

When You Are the Hostess

1 People will expect you to be busy, so I doubt that they will notice if you are eating less in comparison or wonder about it if they do. Don't comment on anybody else's eating habits – they could have a problem they'd rather not broadcast and could be embarrassed by close questioning, however well meant.

2 Never eat something simply because it's there. You aren't starving, and mustn't act as if you'll never get the chance to eat a certain dish ever again. Tell yourself that you can have it any time you want it, but not today. Tell yourself that if you still want it tomorrow, you'll have some then.

The
Maintenance
Diet

I call this my 'free-range' diet because you have more choices. I hope you like it. The meals in the day plans are suggestions. Feel free to eat any of the meals in the recipe section (pages 89–117) instead of ones suggested here.

You are allowed:

- two glasses of wine or champagne every day, or one glass of lager or beer

- bread – slices or rolls – as long as it is unbleached white bread (see recipe on page 114)

- fruit during the day if you wish.

Remember:

- keep salt to a minimum

- portion size is crucial to any weight-loss programme. Use the guidelines on page 40.

Please do not forget that your water intake today and every day should be 2 litres (3½ pints). Drink water during the day at every opportunity.

Day 1

Breakfast Porridge, made with 30g (1oz) oats and water served with a teaspoon of honey, if desired, and skimmed milk
or
Rice Krispies with skimmed milk
or
1 egg, scrambled, on one slice of unbleached white toast

Mid-morning Milky coffee
or
Skimmed milk liquidized with soft fruit and a little sugar if necessary

Lunch Any home-made leaf soup, such as asparagus, spinach or watercress.
Mixed salad with avocado, lean ham or tuna
or
Sliced avocado with either 115g (4oz) prawns and 1 tsp Mayonnaise (page 103) or 2 tbsp hummus
1 slice of unbleached white bread and butter or a roll

Mid-afternoon Small pot live natural yoghurt

Evening meal Grilled fillet of plaice topped with a pat of parsley butter and lemon
Puréed broccoli, carrots
or
Spaghetti Bolognese (page 112)
or
Pasta with Green Vegetable Sauce (page 110)

Dessert Apple or Rhubarb Snow (page 115)
or
Rice Pudding (page 104)

Supper
(if hungry) Handful of grapes
Sliced strawberries
2 flaked almonds or Brazil nuts
Warm milky drink

Day 2

Breakfast

2 slices of unbleached white toast with butter
Cheese spread or Marmite
or
Peeled, stewed apple with 1 dsp fromage frais

Mid-morning

1 banana

Lunch

Cottage cheese and fruit platter, using slices of mango, pineapple and pawpaw or other fruits in season
or
Cold salmon fillet with Dill Cream (from the Fishcakes recipe on page 94 – make double sauce if you are going to have the Fishcakes for your evening meal)
Green salad

Mid-afternoon

Small pot live natural yoghurt

Evening meal

Cheese salad (a colourful mixed salad with red and green peppers, sweet-corn, grated carrot, lettuce and tomatoes, watercress, etc and 30g/1oz grated cheese)
Boiled potatoes
or
Smoked Haddock and Smoked Salmon Fishcakes with Dill Cream (page 94)
Peas
Mashed potato

Dessert

Prunes and apricots
Half-fat crème fraiche or fromage frais or Fresh Custard (page 104)

Supper
(if hungry)

1 apple
A few grapes
A few nuts
Warm milky drink

Day 3

Breakfast Soaked oats, topped with fresh raspberries and yoghurt
or
2 poached eggs
2 rashers bacon, grilled
2 grilled tomatoes

Mid-morning Small pot of cottage cheese with celery sticks

Lunch Spanish Omelette (page 101)
Green salad
or
Cold beef or chicken salad

Mid-afternoon Sliced apple and banana mixed

Evening meal Kedgeree (page 107)
or
Cheese soufflé (page 100)
2 green vegetables

Dessert 6 prunes
6 dried apricots
Half-fat crème fraiche or fromage frais or Fresh Custard (page 104)

Supper
(if hungry) Fruit in season
A few nuts
Warm milky drink

Day 4

Breakfast   Rice Krispies
or
1 boiled egg
1 slice of toast and butter

Mid-morning   Small pot live natural yoghurt

Lunch   2 slices ham
2 sliced tomatoes
Grated carrot and watercress salad
1 roll and butter
or
Avocado and pine nut salad
or
Bacon and egg salad made with 2 slices of bacon, grilled and chopped, 2 hard-boiled eggs, chopped, served on salad leaves with 1 tsp Mayonnaise (page 103)

Mid-afternoon   Glass of skimmed milk
or
Skimmed milk liquidized with soft fruit and a little sugar if necessary

Evening meal   Cod and Prawn Pie (page 106)
Peas and carrots
or
Vegetable Paella (page 109)
or
Coronation Chicken (page 98)
Mixed salad leaves
Basmati rice

Dessert   1 tinned, baked or fresh sliced pear with 1 tbsp Home-Made Chocolate Sauce (page 117)
or
Winter Fruit Salad with yoghurt

Supper
(if hungry)   Fruit in season
A few nuts
Warm milky drink

Day 5

Breakfast	Stay with porridge if you love it
	or
	Rice Krispies
Mid-morning	2 oatcakes with cottage cheese
Lunch	Home-made asparagus or spinach soup
	1 slice of unbleached white bread
	or
	Cold chicken breast
	2 sliced tomatoes
	1 tsp Mayonnaise (page 103)
	Rice
Mid-afternoon	1 banana
Evening meal	Grilled Salmon with Tarragon Butter (page 106)
	Boiled potatoes
	Asparagus or French beans
	or
	Baby Balti Vegetables
	Rice
Dessert	Rice Pudding (page 104)
	or
	Hot Fruit Meringue (page 116)
Supper (if hungry)	Fruit in season
	A few nuts
	Warm milky drink

24-Hour Emergency Plan

What if you've got just a day or so to look your very best? What if you've suddenly been invited somewhere and want to wear your slinkiest outfit or most figure-hugging dress? Do you spend all day nibbling at bits of fruit?

This isn't a weight-loss diet, but when a flatter stomach is particularly important to you it's easy to fall into the trap of eating nothing all day, or snacking on raw vegetables. This isn't the right approach. So what do you do?

1 Start the day before if you can, and for supper have a stir-fry with plenty of sweetcorn, peas and other fresh vegetables. Drink two or three glasses of water during the evening whether you like it or not and have 40g (1$^{1}/_{2}$oz) of All-Bran or bran flakes for supper, with a few grapes, sliced apple and an orange if possible.

2 On the day itself, drink plenty of water. For breakfast have porridge made with 30g (1oz) oats and water served with 1 tsp honey, if desired, and skimmed milk.

3 Throughout the morning, have a tablespoon of live natural yoghurt every hour.

4 For lunch, have a small mixed-leaf salad with chicken or with half an avocado.

5 Two hours later, drink a glass of skimmed milk.

6 In the late afternoon, have a small mixed-leaf salad with 30g (1oz) grated cheese or 2 tablespoons of tuna.

Do not eat after this.
This regime works extremely well for just one day, after which you must go back to normal eating.

Recipes

NO-BLOAT MEALS

The Grenfell programme is about simplicity. Simple meals are not boring meals. By using the freshest and best ingredients you can afford and obtain, you will care for your body holistically. As a result you will find yourself feeling energetic and positive, functioning better, with better skin, a fat-free body and of course that wonderful non-bloated flat stomach.

This section contains standard no-bloat meals. Use them any time you like on the programme. The second section has slightly more ambitious meals which might include a few controversial foods. You might like to save these for non-programme days or you might find your body tolerates the ingredients well.

Whatever you decide to do, you can always add items as it suits you, as long as you remember your basic programme – sitting down to eat, chewing thoroughly and so on.

Cooking Methods

Always poach, grill, stir-fry with minimum oil or roast with a dot of butter. Never deep-fry or boil out of existence!

Basic Fish Meals

Cod, Halibut, Haddock, Etc.

On the 5-Day programme, white fish should be poached in milk or water and served plain on a bed of:

- spinach (cod or plaice Florentine)
- mashed carrots
- mashed parsnips.

White fish can also be baked in the oven in a sauce of tinned, chopped tomatoes with, say, sliced bottled sweet red pimentos (found in all supermarkets in vegetable section).

Cod in Parsley Sauce

Bake a 140g (5oz) portion of cod in enough skimmed milk to cover.

For the sauce

1 dsp cornflour

2 dsp cold milk

small bunch flat-leaf parsley, chopped finely

salt and freshly ground black pepper

In a saucepan, mix the cornflour and cold milk to a paste. Warm through.

Add the strained, cooked milk from the fish and bring to a simmer, stirring constantly, until the sauce begins to thicken.

Remove from the heat immediately and stir in the parsley.

Season to taste.

Place the cod on a serving plate and cover with the sauce.

Salade Niçoise

This is a standard tuna fish salad, with hard-boiled egg, cold French beans and a sprinkling of olives. Layer the salad starting with lettuce, lamb's lettuce and watercress. Add the other ingredients, finishing with 100g (3½oz) tuna fish.

Feel free to add ingredients as they suit you. Lemon juice or Vinaigrette (page 103) are suitable dressings, or use the Dill Cream from the Fishcakes recipe on page 94.

Salmon

Salmon with Almond and Honey Crust

Making this dish is like battering a piece of fish!

Serves 2

2 salmon fillets

2 tsp butter

2 tsp runny honey

1 dsp skinless flaked almonds, crushed roughly

Preheat the oven to 200ºC/400ºF/gas mark 6.

Put the butter and honey in a heatproof ramekin and heat through or microwave until melted and runny.

Place the crushed almonds on a flat plate.

Pat the salmon dry. Dip it into, or brush with, the butter and honey mixture, top side only.

Now firmly press the buttered side of the fish onto the crushed almonds and pour over any remaining butter mixture.

Place in a greased, ovenproof dish or a throwaway foil tray. Cover with foil and bake for 15 minutes. Then remove the foil to allow the top crust of the fish to crisp (5 minutes).

Sesame or Pine Nut Salmon with Orange

Serves 4

packet of pine nuts or 4 tbsp sesame seeds

2 oranges, washed

4 salmon fillets

1 tbsp butter, melted

Preheat the oven to 200°C/400°F/gas mark 6.

Scatter the sesame seeds or pine nuts over a dinner plate with the pared rind of one of the oranges. Squeeze both oranges and reserve the juice.

Pat the salmon fillets dry and brush them with melted butter. Place butter-side down on the seeds or nuts and orange. Press thoroughly to coat each side. Put in an ovenproof dish and pour the orange juice over.

Bake for 20 minutes.

Barbecued Salmon with Citrus

Serves 4

1–2 oranges

30g (1oz) butter, preferably unsalted

2 tbsp chopped dill

2 cloves garlic, crushed

salt and freshly ground black pepper

1 x 900g (2lb) piece middle-cut salmon

Cut off the tops and bottoms of the oranges, then cut in half from top to bottom and slice.

Mix the butter, dill and garlic together and season. Put two large sheets of foil one on top of the other.

Stuff the salmon with half the butter mixture and half the orange slices. Spread half the remaining butter over one half of the foil and arrange half the orange slices on it.

Place the salmon on top of the butter and fruit slices. Spread the remaining butter over the top of the fish and arrange the remaining orange slices on it.

Bring the unbuttered side of the foil over the fish and make a loose parcel with the join on one side. Seal well.

Make three 5–7.5cm (2–3 inch) angled slashes in the foil on both sides. Place on a rack over a good quantity of glowing coals. Keep the coals very hot and cook for 20 minutes on each side. To test if cooked, partly open the parcel. Use a fork to check that the salmon flesh easily comes away from the bone.

Smoked Haddock and Smoked Salmon Fishcakes with Dill Cream

Serves 2

1 cup skimmed milk

2 large fillets skinless and boneless smoked haddock

2 large potatoes

2 slices smoked salmon or 100g (3½oz) smoked
 salmon offcuts or cubes

20g (¾oz) butter

freshly ground black pepper

1 tbsp fresh parsley, chopped

flour for dusting

For the dill cream

1 tsp snipped fresh dill or ½ tsp dried dill

1 tbsp Mayonnaise (page 103)

1 tbsp half-fat crème fraiche.

Preheat the oven to 180°C/350°F/gas mark 4.

Put the milk in an ovenproof dish together with the haddock. Poach in the oven for 20 minutes.

Meanwhile, peel and boil the potatoes. Drain and mash without butter or milk.

Turn the oven up to 220°C/450°F/gas mark 7.

Place the poached haddock in a large bowl, reserving the milk first. Mash roughly with a fork, keeping some large flakes of fish.

Chop and add the smoked salmon, the mashed potato, half of the butter, black pepper to taste and the parsley. Mix thoroughly.

Using floured hands, shape the fishcakes into rounds. If the mixture is stiff, add a little of the milk the fish was poached in. You should make about eight fishcakes.

Place fishcakes on a greased baking sheet, using a little butter. Dot the remainder of the butter on the fishcakes.

Place in the hot oven for 20–30 minutes, turning once.

To make the dill cream

Mix the mayonnaise, crème fraiche and snipped dill.

To serve, place a teaspoon of the dill cream on each fishcake and save the rest.

Save the four fishcakes you did not use – you can reheat them the following day.

Chicken

Grilled Chicken in Orange Marinade

Serves 1

120–150g (4–5oz) skinless, boneless chicken breast

juice and zest of 1 large orange

1 tbsp walnut oil or olive oil

1 clove garlic, crushed (optional)

Place all the ingredients in an ovenproof dish, stir well to mix, cover with foil and refrigerate overnight if possible, or for at least two hours.

Preheat the oven to 180°C/350°F/gas mark 4. Remove the chicken from the dish and place on a wire rack over a roasting tin in the oven. Cook for about 20 minutes.

Turn the grill to high, and grill the chicken thoroughly on both sides until brown and slightly caramelized.

Alternatively pan-fry with the lid on tightly, over medium heat, turning frequently to prevent burning. This takes about 10 minutes.

Chicken with a Pine Nut Crust

Serves 4

4 boneless chicken breasts

packet of pine nuts

oil

Flatten 4 boneless chicken breasts with a rolling pin, after covering the chicken with a piece of greaseproof paper. This avoids tearing the meat.

Scatter a packet of pine nuts over a dinner plate. Brush the chicken breasts with oil and place on the pine nuts. Press thoroughly to coat each side.

Fry gently in a pan containing 1 tbsp oil, turning once.

Alternatively you can preheat the oven to 200°C/400°F/gas mark 6 and cook on a rack for 20 minutes.

Coconut Chicken Curry

Serves 4

2 tsp oil

1 stalk lemon grass, trimmed and chopped

1 heaped tsp fresh shredded ginger

3 tbsp green curry paste

6 kaffir lime leaves, if available

4 chicken breast fillets, halved and flattened

570ml (1 pint) coconut milk

handful basil leaves

handful coriander leaves

Heat the oil in a saucepan over medium heat. Add the lemon grass and ginger and cook for 4 minutes.

Add the curry paste and shredded lime leaves and cook, stirring, for 2 minutes.

Add the chicken and coconut milk to the pan and allow to simmer for 20 minutes. Stir in the basil and coriander.

Chicken Roulade with Spinach

Serves 2

2 medium chicken breasts (about 140g/5oz each)

bag of young spinach leaves (about 50–100g/2–4oz
according to taste)

2 tsp butter

2 tbsp half-fat crème fraiche

nutmeg

salt and freshly ground black pepper

1 dsp oil

You will also need some string.

Make a slit along the side of each chicken breast, open out and flatten with a rolling pin beneath grease-proof paper. Alternatively, buy chicken escalopes and flatten until quite thin.

Very slightly wilt the spinach by heating 1 tsp butter in a lidded pan with 1 dsp water. Add the spinach and put the lid on tight. Shake the pan gently over a high heat for about 20 seconds until the spinach has wilted. Cool.

Place a mound of spinach on the chicken escalope and spread out. Then roll the chicken up, making sure the spinach does not escape. It should resemble a Swiss roll.

Tie each escalope loosely with string at 2–3cm (1 inch) intervals, to prevent it unrolling.

Place in a frying pan with a little oil. Gently fry, turning frequently, for about ten minutes. Make sure it is cooked through, not pink inside. Do not brown.

When thoroughly cooked (test with a knife – the flesh should be white throughout without a hint of pink) add the crème fraiche to the pan. Heat through, season to taste with nutmeg, salt and pepper. Remove the chicken roulades reserving the cream sauce.

Slice each roulade into tiny rounds. They should resemble Swiss rolls with the green filling showing throughout in a spiral. Spoon over the crème fraiche.

Spicy, Yoghurt-Baked Chicken

Serves 2

1 small carton (120–150g/4–5$\frac{1}{2}$oz) natural live bio
yoghurt

juice of 1 fresh lime

a little fresh ginger root, grated

few fennel seeds

1 tsp each ground cumin, turmeric and cayenne
pepper

1 clove garlic, crushed (optional)

2 chicken breasts

To prepare the marinade, combine the yoghurt, lime juice, spices and garlic in a bowl and mix thoroughly.

Place the chicken in the marinade, coat completely, cover and set aside for 2–8 hours.

Preheat the oven to 180°C/350°F/gas mark 4.

Place the chicken in an ovenproof dish and cook in the oven for 25 minutes. Spread the rest of the marinade over the chicken and return to the oven uncovered for about 30 minutes.

Serve with basmati rice and a green salad.

Coronation Chicken

Serves 1

1 tsp apricot jam

½ tbsp Mayonnaise (page 103)

1–2 tsp curry powder

few flaked almonds (optional)

1 small chicken breast (6oz/170g), roasted, cooled
   and cut into strips

Mix the jam, mayonnaise, curry powder, almonds and
chicken. Combine thoroughly. Add more curry powder
if you like it spicy.

   Serve on a bed of mixed salad leaves with basmati
rice.

Chicken Malibu Salad

Serves 4

4 chicken breasts

1 large cos lettuce, chopped

1 bunch mint

170g (6oz) blueberries

For the dressing

300ml (½ pint) Greek yoghurt

1 tsp brown sugar

1 tsp ground cumin

juice of 1 lemon

1 tbsp olive oil

Grill or charcoal grill the chicken breasts and arrange
down the centre of a serving plate.

   Combine all the dressing ingredients in a bowl and
beat well. Stir in most of the blueberries, reserving a
few to scatter garnish.

   Surround the chicken with the lettuce and mint
sprigs.

   Spoon the dressing generously over the chicken
and scatter with the blueberries and chopped mint.

Vegetarian

Caesar Salad v

Serves 2

1 tbsp Mayonnaise (page 103)

1 garlic clove, crushed

1 slice thick-cut stale bread

vegetable oil

1 cos lettuce, separated into leaves

30g (1oz) Parmesan cheese, coarsely grated

Mix the garlic into the mayonnaise.

   Make the croutons by cutting the bread into half-inch cubes. Heat the oil until very hot and fry the cubes quickly until golden brown, which will take a couple of minutes. Remove with a slotted spoon and blot dry with kitchen paper.

   Add the cooled croutons and the mayonnaise to the lettuce and toss together. Sprinkle the Parmesan cheese over the salad and serve.

Cheese Soufflé ν

Soufflés are not nearly as difficult or exacting to make as people think, and I have often guessed at the quantities, thrown them all in and still had a sensational result.

Serves 2

15g (½oz) self-raising flour

150ml (¼ pint) skimmed milk

3 large eggs, separated

   (you will use only two of the yolks)

60g (2oz) strong Cheddar, Leicester or Cheshire

   cheese, finely grated

15g (½oz) Parmesan cheese, grated (optional)

salt and freshly ground black pepper

Preheat the oven to 200°C/400°F/gas mark 6.

Grease a medium soufflé dish and tie a piece of greaseproof paper round the outside to hold the soufflé as it rises.

In a saucepan, mix the flour with a little cold milk to form a smooth paste. Gently bring to a simmer, gradually adding the rest of the milk and stirring all the time as it thickens.

Allow the sauce to cool slightly. Cover the pan to make sure that it does not form a skin.

Add the two egg yolks and beat the mixture until it is smooth.

Add the cheese and seasoning.

Whisk the three egg whites until stiff but not dry. Add the cheese and sauce mixture to the egg whites – not the other way round. Do this gently so you don't knock the air out of the whites.

Transfer immediately to the soufflé dish and bake for about 15–20 minutes, or until golden brown on top.

Eat immediately with a green salad.

Spinach Soufflé ν

Serves 2

1 tbsp cornflour

300ml (½ pint) semi-skimmed milk

4 large eggs, separated

500g (1lb) mashed spinach, cooked with a dot of

   butter, salt and freshly ground black pepper

small tub cottage cheese (optional, but gives extra

   flavour)

Preheat the oven to 200°C/400°F/gas mark 6.

Grease a large soufflé dish or ovenproof, straight-sided dish.

In a saucepan, mix the cornflour with a little cold milk to form a smooth paste. Gently bring to a simmer, gradually adding the rest of the milk and stirring all the time as it thickens.

Allow the sauce to cool slightly. Cover the pan to make sure that it does not form a skin.

Beat the egg yolks into the sauce one at a time. It should become smooth and shiny. Add the mashed spinach and cottage cheese if using.

Whisk the egg whites in a large bowl until stiff but not dry.

Add the sauce to the egg whites – not the other way round. Do this gently so you don't knock the air out of the whites. Combine carefully, then turn immediately into the soufflé dish.

Cook for about 20–30 minutes, or until the top has separated slightly and formed a golden crust.

Eat immediately.

Herb, Cheese or Spanish Omelette *V*

All types of omelette are good non-bloat dishes. Use three eggs per person and 1 tsp of butter in the pan. For a herb omelette, add a mixture of herbs to taste. For a cheese omelette, add 15g (½oz) grated Cheddar cheese.

For a Spanish omelette, add chopped red and green pepper and a few chunks of cold potato.

Spinach omelettes are also good.

Herb Omelette Salad *V*

Serves 4

4 eggs, beaten

2 tbsp chopped fresh herbs

Salt and freshly ground black pepper

Butter

1 large red pepper, seeded and cut into strips

1 large green pepper, seeded and cut into strips

½ cucumber, cut into thin strips

Vinaigrette (page 103) to taste

Beat the eggs with the herbs and 2 tbsp water. Season with salt and pepper. Heat a knob of butter or margarine in an omelette pan and use the eggs to make two thinly, lightly set omelettes. Turn out on to a sheet of greaseproof paper, roll up and leave to cool slightly.

Toss the remaining ingredients together.

Thinly slice the omelette and scatter over the prepared salad ingredients. Serve immediately.

Baked Cheese Tomatoes *V*

Serves 1

30g (1oz) grated mature Cheddar cheese

2 large beef tomatoes

Preheat the oven to 180°C/350°F/gas mark 4.

Simply scoop out the middle of the tomatoes and discard the seeds. Fill the cavity with the grated cheese, half in each tomato.

Using a sharp knife, score through the skin right round the tomato. This will stop the skin splitting.

Bake for 10–15 minutes or grill until the cheese is bubbling and slightly browned.

Beef

On the 5-Day programme you are always
permitted a small fillet or sirloin steak with salad
or spinach. For your evening meals, you may also
have other mixed vegetables, especially parsnips,
carrots, Swede and courgettes, marrows,
mangetout, sugar snap peas and French beans.

Sauces and Dressings

Vinaigrette (French Dressing)

This keeps for ages in the fridge. The amount you make is up to you, depending on whether you are in a single household or are feeding half a dozen. The proportions are the same:

Use 3 parts olive oil or good vegetable oil to one part wine vinegar.

Pour into a screw-top jar.

Add 2 tsp Dijon mustard, 1 tsp sugar and some coarsely ground black pepper.

If you like garlic, add a crushed clove.

Shake the mixture thoroughly and taste. Adjust to suit your own tastes.

Mayonnaise

Most people who are dieting worry unnecessarily about the high oil content in mayonnaise. The first consideration is that in fresh mayonnaise most of the fat content is good fat – not saturated – and the second is that we use tiny quantities. Use this mayonnaise on your hard-boiled eggs or your cold poached salmon. It will last for up to two days in the fridge. Use either a blender or an electric whisk for this.

1 egg yolk (reserve the white for something else, like cheese soufflé or a meringue)

570ml (1 pint) good oil

Place the egg yolk in a clean bowl and add a few drops of oil, whisking all the time. Continue to add the oil by the drop until it seems that the mixture is amalgamating.

Graduate to pouring the oil in a thin stream. But slowly – if you start to pour the oil too quickly, the mixture will curdle.

Continue pouring, mixing all the time, until the mixture is thick and creamy.

If the mixture curdles, try rescuing it by adding a spoonful of hot water or a small dash of vinegar. If you have spoilt it, however, start again with a fresh yolk and add the curdled mixture, bit by bit.

Now you have a basic mayonnaise. Try a teaspoon of curry powder for curried mayonnaise (great for Coronation Chicken, page 98) or the grated zest of a lemon for lemon mayonnaise. Or add some crushed garlic or finely chopped basil leaves.

Desserts

Fresh Custard

Your own custard is so easy to make, I don't know why people don't make it more often. You can keep it in the fridge for a couple of days. A piece of cling film laid on the surface will stop a skin forming.

1 egg yolk (reserve the white for something else, like
    cheese soufflé or a meringue)

1¹/₂ tbsp caster sugar

1 tsp cornflour

300ml (¹/₂ pint) skimmed milk

vanilla essence

In a small jug, mix the egg yolk with the sugar and cornflour to make a smooth paste. Add a little cold milk.

Put the rest of the milk in a pan and heat through. When it is coming to the boil, remove from the heat and add a little to the egg mixture, stirring all the time. Pour back into the pan and keep stirring over a low heat while the custard thickens. Add a few drops of vanilla essence.

If the custard curdles, which may happen if it gets too hot, pour it into a cold bowl and whisk.

Rice Pudding

Serves 3–4

I first became enthusiastic about rice pudding when I was pregnant with my second child and had to endure a long journey from the country to town and a freezing mile walk to the hospital for my check-ups. The whole procedure took half a day, but by starting with porridge and taking a pot of rice pudding with me I managed it with gusto – not easy when you're trailing a two-year-old.

Since then I have made a rice pudding every week, summer or winter, because it is not only nourishing and healthy but it is equally delicious hot or cold. The calorie content is not at all high for a snack, and with the addition of stewed fruit, you will have no need of another meal. Made with skimmed milk it's full of calcium, protein and starch. Try it!

60g (2oz) short-grain (pudding) rice

570ml (1 pint) skimmed milk

1¹/₂ tbsp sugar

Preheat the oven to 180˚C/350˚F/gas mark 4.

Combine all the ingredients in a lightly greased pudding basin and cook for 2 hours, stirring occasion-ally to separate rice grains.

Either eat straight away, hot, with a teaspoon of jam in the middle, or cool completely, decant into 3–4 empty yoghurt pots and refrigerate until needed. It can then be microwaved if you want it hot.

MAINTENANCE PROGRAMME RECIPES

Once again, these 'recipes' are more like cooking methods.
The ingredients are simple but delicious.

Grilled Salmon with Tarragon Butter

Serves 1

1 125–180g (4–6oz) salmon fillet

1 tsp butter

fresh tarragon leaves, chopped, or a pinch of dried
  tarragon

parsley to garnish

Grill the fish with a dot of the butter.

Soften the rest of the butter, combine with the tarragon and place it on the hot fish.

Garnish with parsley and serve immediately with vegetables.

Cod and Prawn Pie

Serves 2

360ml ($^3/_4$ pint) skimmed milk

225g (8oz) cod fillet, or two frozen portions, thawed

450g (1lb) old potatoes, peeled and diced

handful of broccoli florets, broken into small pieces

30g (1oz) cornflour

1 tsp mustard powder

salt and freshly ground black pepper

sprig of fresh parsley, chopped

60g (2oz) Cheddar cheese, grated

115g (4oz) frozen prawns, thawed and drained

Put half the milk into a small frying pan and add the cod, whole. Cover and bring to a gentle simmer on a very low heat. Poach gently until cooked through (about 8–10 minutes). Drain and reserve the liquid.

Break the fish into large chunks or flakes and put into a shallow ovenproof casserole dish. Preheat the oven to 180°C/350°F/gas mark 4.

Boil the potatoes. Boil or steam the broccoli for 3 minutes. Drain and reserve.

Make a sauce by putting the milk the fish was poached in into a saucepan and heating gently. Mix the cornflour with a tablespoon of cool milk until it forms a smooth paste. Add the paste to the milk in the pan and raise the heat slightly, stirring constantly as the mixture thickens to avoid burning or lumps forming.

Take off the heat and add the mustard powder, seasoning and parsley. Stir in the cheese and beat gently as the cheese melts.

Drain the potatoes and mash with the remaining milk.

Arrange the broccoli over the cod chunks, add the prawns and pour on the cheese sauce.

Spoon the mashed potato over the top or pipe in swirls if you want a more dressy appearance.

Cook in the oven for 20–30 minutes, or until the top is golden.

Kedgeree

Serves 2

Served as a main meal with a green salad or other vegetables, this makes a slightly exotic, very nourishing and tasty meal. Alternatively, served as a light lunch dish, or traditionally as a breakfast dish, you can halve the quantities given here. Better still, train yourself to eat less – try having half now and half later.

2 fillets smoked haddock, about 225g (8oz) each

1 cup skimmed milk to poach

100g (3½oz) basmati rice

1 tsp butter

½ an onion, finely chopped

1–2 tsp mild curry powder

1 tsp turmeric

pinch cayenne pepper

nutmeg

2 hard-boiled eggs, shelled and cut into quarters

freshly ground black pepper

Place the haddock in a pan, cover with the milk and set to poach gently for about 8 minutes until softened through.

Meanwhile, cook the rice, following the directions on the packet.

In separate pan, melt the butter and gently fry the onion until soft.

Add the drained rice, curry powder, turmeric, cayenne pepper and nutmeg to the onion and stir.

Flake the cooked haddock, reserving the cooking milk. Add the fish to the rice mixture.

Add the eggs and milk to the rice and fish mixture.

Season if necessary, stir and serve hot.

Warm Chicken and Potato Salad

Serves 4

2 tbsp olive oil

1kg (2lb 2oz) tiny new potatoes, halved

4 bacon rashers, roughly chopped

meat of 1 large cooked chicken or 3 cooked chicken breasts, cooked.

2 tbsp soured cream

1 tbsp Mayonnaise (page 103)

2 tsp seeded mustard

¼ cup finely chopped fresh chives

Preheat the oven to 230°C/450°F/gas mark 8. Combine the oil and potatoes in a large baking dish and bake, uncovered, for 25 minutes, turning once during cooking.

Meanwhile, cook the bacon in a large heated pan until crisp and drain on absorbent paper. Remove and discard any skin and bones from the chicken and chop the meat roughly.

Gently toss the cooked potatoes, bacon and chicken in a large bowl with the soured cream, mayonnaise, mustard and chives.

Serve on a bed of salad leaves.

Italia Grape and Chicken Salad

Serves 4

450g (1lb) Italia green grapes, deseeded

450g (1lb) cooked cold chicken, cut into bite-sized
    pieces

1 pack mixed salad leaves

1 tbsp pine kernels, toasted

fresh basil leaves to garnish

For the dressing

4 tbsp half-fat crème fraiche

3 tbsp olive oil

1 tbsp pesto

1 tbsp lemon juice

salt and freshly ground black pepper

Place the grapes and chicken in a large bowl.

Whisk the dressing ingredients together in a bowl
until well blended. Pour the dressing over the grapes
and chicken and toss together.

Arrange the salad leaves in a shallow salad bowl
and pile the grape and chicken mixture in the centre.
Scatter the pine kernels over it and garnish with basil
leaves.

Courgette, Carrot, Grapefruit and Avocado Salad V

Serves 2

1 avocado

1–2 carrots, scraped

2 large courgettes

1 grapefruit

Vinaigrette (page 103)

coarsely ground black pepper

Cut the avocado in two and discard the stone. Cut
away the outer shell and slice each half in strips.

Using a potato peeler, slice long strips down the
length of the carrots and courgettes, making ribbons.

Cut the grapefruit in two halves and, preferably
using a grapefruit knife, carefully cut out segments.
Add to the vegetables.

Add enough Vinaigrette to coat the vegetables.
Sprinkle with black pepper.

Vegetable Paella V

Serves 2

$^1/_2$ an aubergine, chopped

salt

1 tbsp olive oil

$^1/_2$ a small onion, chopped

3 slices each red and green pepper, chopped

$^1/_2$ a carrot, chopped

1 clove garlic, crushed

100g (3$^1/_2$oz) long-grain rice

1 small tin of chopped tomatoes with herbs

$^1/_2$ tsp turmeric

coarsely ground black pepper

fresh parsley

Lay the aubergine on a board and cover with salt. Leave for 20 minutes. Wash and drain.

Heat the olive oil in a large frying pan. Add the onions and gently sauté until soft.

Add the peppers, aubergine, carrot and garlic, and stir.

Add the raw rice and the tomatoes, plus 300ml ($^1/_2$ pint) water and the turmeric. Season to taste.

Bring to the boil, then reduce heat and simmer until all the water has been absorbed by the rice.

Serve with a good sprinkling of parsley.

Baby Balti Vegetables V

Serves 2

There are a wide variety of baby vegetables available these days, usually aimed at the stir-fry market. This simple recipe can be prepared very quickly with little equipment.

8 baby new potatoes

8 baby carrots

6 baby courgettes

2 tbsp corn oil

8 baby onions, peeled

1 tsp root ginger, grated

1 garlic clove, crushed

1 tbsp chilli sauce

115g (4oz) cooked chickpeas or 1 small can

handful of mangetouts

8 baby corn

8 cherry tomatoes

1 tsp dried chillies

$^3/_4$ tbsp sesame seeds

Bring a pan of water to the boil and add the potatoes and the carrots. After 5–8 minutes (depending on the size of the vegetables) add the courgettes and boil for a further two minutes. Drain and reserve.

Heat the oil in a large frying pan or wok. Add the onions and fry until golden brown. Lower the heat and add the ginger, garlic and chilli sauce.

Add the chickpeas and stir-fry over a medium heat until all the moisture has been absorbed.

Add the cooked potatoes, carrots and courgettes, plus the mangetouts, baby corn and tomatoes. Stir over the heat for a further 2 minutes.

Add the crushed chillies, turn onto a serving plate and sprinkle with the sesame seeds.

Serve with basmati rice or nan bread.

Smoked Salmon with Pasta, Watercress and Dill

Serves 1

60g (2oz) dry pasta shapes

1 slice smoked salmon cut into strips (or about
   100g/3$\frac{1}{2}$oz ready sliced)

few fronds of snipped fresh dill or a pinch of dried dill

1 large bunch watercress, stems removed

freshly ground black pepper

1 dsp half-fat crème fraiche

Boil the pasta until cooked. Drain and return to the
pan.

Keeping the heat under the pan very low, add the
smoked salmon and stir through quickly. The salmon
will go pale as it cooks.

Straight away, add the dill and watercress. Mix
thoroughly, then add the crème fraiche and black pepper. Taste for seasoning. (The salmon is very salty, so
don't add any salt.)

Serve immediately on very hot plates, as pasta
goes cold very quickly.

Pasta with Green Vegetable Sauce V

Serves 2–3

**This sauce can be made with frozen broad beans
and peas, but is best in the summer when the fresh
vegetables come into season.**

170g (6oz) dried pasta shapes

100g (3$\frac{1}{2}$oz) broad beans, boiled and cooled

100g (3$\frac{1}{2}$oz) fresh peas, boiled and cooled

12 asparagus tips (optional, and tinned will do)

1 courgette, sliced, with skin on

2 tbsp walnut or sunflower oil

2 large tbsp half-fat crème fraiche

a few fresh tarragon leaves, chopped, or $\frac{1}{2}$ tsp dried
   tarragon

salt and freshly ground black pepper

a bunch of fresh parsley, chopped

a few shavings fresh Parmesan cheese

Boil the pasta according to directions on the packet.
Drain and reserve.

While the pasta is cooking, stir-fry all the vegetables in the oil for about 2–3 minutes in a large frying
pan. Make sure you slightly sear the courgette and
asparagus.

Add the cooked pasta shapes and mix together to
heat through. Add the crème fraiche and, keeping the
heat low, stir through to heat gently without curdling.
Finally, add the herbs and season.

Turn out onto hot plates (pasta goes cold very
quickly), top with the parsley and the Parmesan
cheese.

Spaghetti Alla Carbonara

Serves 2

I first experienced this dish in 1970 when staying with an Italian friend in her cramped bedsit in London. With only a single gas ring to cook on, she showed me how to conjure up this magnificent dish in twenty minutes, now reduced to ten minutes by the widespread availability of fresh pasta. I have adapted it slightly for slimming purposes, but remember that we eat smaller portions anyway!

2 rashers smoked back bacon

100g (3½oz) fresh spaghetti

1 egg yolk

coarsely ground black pepper

2 tbsp single cream

a splash of good olive oil

Using a standard saucepan or frying pan, fry the bacon without fat until well cooked. Set aside.

Bring a large pan of water to the boil and add the spaghetti. Time it to simmer for three minutes.

While the spaghetti is cooking, chop the bacon into pieces.

Mix the egg yolk, pepper and cream in a cup.

After three minutes, drain the spaghetti thoroughly and return to the pan, keeping the heat low.

Add the olive oil, bacon bits, egg-and-cream mixture and toss. Turn off the heat and continue stirring. (If you leave the heat on the eggs start to scramble.)

Serve immediately on a very hot plate (pasta goes cold very quickly).

Pasta Primavera V

Serves 1

60g (2oz) fresh pasta spirals or penne

1 tbsp olive oil

handful of mangetouts, baby corn, sugar snap peas, carrot sticks, red and green peppers, bean sprouts

1 tsp pesto sauce

2 tsp half-fat crème fraiche

salt and freshly ground black pepper

Cook the pasta according to the instructions on the packet. Drain and keep warm.

In a deep frying pan or wok, heat the oil and add the mixed vegetables. Toss over a high heat for one minute.

Add the drained pasta and the pesto sauce. Turn for thirty seconds.

Remove from heat, add the crème fraiche, stir, check seasoning and serve immediately on a hot plate.

Spaghetti Bolognese

Serves 2

225g (8oz) extra-lean mince

1½ tbsp olive oil

1 small onion, finely chopped

1 clove garlic, crushed (optional)

225g (8oz) tinned chopped tomatoes with herbs

1 tbsp concentrated tomato purée

225g (8oz) fresh spaghetti

few leaves fresh oregano or ½ tsp dried oregano

salt and freshly ground black pepper

Parmesan cheese

In a large frying pan, fry the mince without added fat or oil until any fat runs clear. Drain. Set the meat aside.

Heat the oil and gently sauté the onion until softened. Drain off any excess oil and add the mince, garlic, tomatoes and tomato paste. Turn down the heat, cover the pan and simmer for 5 minutes.

Cook the spaghetti as directed on the packet.

Add the oregano to the mince mixture. Stir and taste. Season if necessary. Drain the spaghetti and add the mince mixture to the pasta and toss.

Sprinkle with Parmesan cheese and serve with a green salad.

Beef

On the Maintenance programme, you may have a small fillet or sirloin steak with salad and other vegetables, including parsnips, carrots, Swede and courgettes, marrows, mangetout, sugar snap peas and French beans and a portion of potatoes.

Boeuf Bourguignon

Serves 4

This dish is not the traditional, standard French dish, but it is a good Grenfell-style alternative. I have removed the onion and mushrooms. It still tastes excellent, mostly thanks to the bacon and brandy. Serve with crisp green vegetables from the list of those allowed or with young new potatoes or rice.

1 dsp vegetable oil

700g (1½lb) best stewing or braising steak, cubed
    (use e.g. Aberdeen Angus or leanest braising beef)

1 glass brandy

½ bottle cheap red wine

½ clove garlic, crushed (optional)

6 rashers best back bacon, smoked

1 tbsp cornflour

2 tins chopped tomatoes with added herbs and olives

4 dsp tomato purée

seasonings, to taste: salt, freshly ground black pepper, fresh herbs

fresh parsley (preferably flat-leaf)

2 tbsp half-fat crème fraiche

Preheat the oven to 170°C/325°F/gas mark 3.

Heat the oil over a moderate heat in a large pan, and add the cubed beef. Keep turning to seal all sides, until all traces of red have gone.

Add the brandy, turn heat high and allow to 'flame'. Turn down the heat and add the wine and crushed garlic (if using), plus 2 glasses of water. Stir.

Transfer to a casserole dish, put the lid on tightly and cook in the oven for 1½ hours.

Meanwhile, chop and fry the bacon and set aside. When cool, toss in 1 tbsp cornflour and stir to coat. Save.

When the beef comes out of the oven, add the tinned tomatoes and tomato purée. Mix well. Stir in the bacon. Return to the oven for 1 hour.

Remove from the oven and stir well. Add a little more water if needed, but do not make the casserole too wet.

Taste – you might like to add a little salt, pepper and mixed herbs, to taste.

Return to the oven to heat through. Just before –serving, stir in 2 tbsp half-fat crème fraiche and top with a good sprinkling of coarsely chopped fresh parsley.

Shepherd's Pie

Serves 2

225g (8oz) extra-lean mince

1 beef stock cube

225g (8oz) potatoes, peeled and sliced

1 small onion, finely chopped

4 carrots, finely chopped

1 tsp butter

50ml (2fl oz) skimmed milk

1 tbsp gravy powder

salt and freshly ground black pepper

Preheat the oven to 180°C/350°F/gas mark 4.

In a large frying pan, fry the mince without added fat or oil until any fat runs clear. Drain and put the mince in a large saucepan. Add the stock cube, dissolved as directed, and leave to simmer for 10 minutes.

Boil the potatoes until soft. Then drain them and mash with the butter and milk. Leave to cool slightly.

Add the onion and carrots to the mince.

In a cup, mix the gravy powder with a little water until smooth. Add to the mince, stirring all the time. Put the mince in an ovenproof dish, season to taste and top with the mashed potato.

Cook until brown on top.

Serve with green vegetables.

Unbleached White Bread

Makes one large or two small loaves

500g (1lb 2oz) unbleached organic white flour

1 sachet easy-bake yeast

1 tsp salt

2 tsp sugar

1 tbsp olive oil or 1 tsp butter

340ml (12fl oz) warm water with 2 tbsp milk

Sift the flour into a large bowl, make a well in the centre and add the water, milk, yeast, sugar, salt and oil or butter.

Fold the flour over the top and start to incorporate the ingredients. The mixture might feel sticky to start with, but it will soon start to combine.

If the mixture is a little wet, add more flour, a teaspoon at a time.

Once the dough has formed into a ball, turn it onto a floured surface to begin kneading.

Knead the dough, repeatedly bringing the outside to the centre, for at least ten minutes; this is hard work, but worth it. When it is ready, put back into your mixing bowl and cover with a clean tea towel to rise. This will take about two hours at room temperature, or you can leave it overnight in the fridge. Don't leave it somewhere too warm – this will kill the yeast.

When the dough has doubled in size, take it out and knead again. This is called 'knocking-back' as all the air will go out of it. Do not knead again fully; simply place dough into one large or two smaller greased and floured bread tins. Cover and leave in a warm place, to rise again.

Preheat the oven to 220°C/425°F/gas mark 7. When the bread dough has doubled in size once again, you are ready to bake your bread.

Bake for 20–30 minutes, or until the bread sounds hollow when tapped on the bottom. If it is not ready, put it back into the oven on the bare shelf, not in the tin, for a few minutes.

Allow to cool completely before slicing.

Desserts

Fruit Snow

Serves 2–3

You can make this with any fruit. It is especially good with apple and blackberries, strawberries or raspberries, rhubarb and gooseberries, and is handy for using up a glut of fruit you may have frozen since the summer.

1 egg white

30g (1oz) caster sugar

225g (8oz) fruit, stewed to a purée

Whisk the egg white until stiff, then fold in the sugar and whisk again until shiny and very stiff.

Add the fruit purée to the egg white – not the other way round – fold together gently.

Serve immediately. This looks wonderful in tall glasses.

Winter Fruit Salad

Serves 2

300ml (½ pint) pure apple juice

strip of orange zest

1 cinnamon stick

a few cloves

175g (6oz) mixed dried fruit (prunes, peaches, apricots)

115g (4oz) blackberries

1 pear

1 tbsp brandy (optional)

1 tbsp half-fat crème fraiche or fromage frais or Fresh
   Custard (page 104) (optional)

Put the apple juice, orange zest, cinnamon stick,
cloves and fruit into a pan and heat through on a very
low heat until the mixture is simmering gently. Simmer
for 20 minutes or until the fruit is soft.

Remove from the heat and stir in the brandy,
if using.

Serve warm or cool with the crème fraiche,
fromage frais or custard, if desired.

Hot Fruit Meringue

Serves 3–4

Hot fruit meringues are a simple way of serving a
nice hot pudding in the winter without all the fuss
of a pie or crumble, and certainly without all the
calories. Although apple and blackberry, rhubarb or
plain apple are the usual bases, I have also used
combinations including banana and strawberry or
apricot, prune and blackberry. Stew the fruit in the
usual way, making enough to fill a small ovenproof
dish by two-thirds.

2 or 3 egg whites

60g (2 oz) caster sugar

stewed fruit, cooled

Preheat the oven to 180°C/350°F/gas mark 4.

Whisk the egg whites until stiff. Fold in the sugar
and whisk again.

Spoon the egg over the cooled fruit mixture and
use it to seal the edges of the dish to prevent the fruit
'boiling over'.

Bake for about 10–15 minutes, or until golden
brown on top. Serve hot.

Home-Made Chocolate Sauce

I don't use a lot of this, but a spoonful over half
a tinned or baked pear makes a delicious and sur-
prisingly low-calorie sweet dish. Don't make too
much, or you'll be tempted to dip into it!

225g (8oz) block dark plain chocolate

360ml (³/₄ pint) water

60g (2oz) caster sugar

100ml (3¹/₂fl oz) double cream

Put the chocolate into the water, in a pan.
    Add the sugar. Bring to the boil and reduce to
a simmer for 15 minutes.
    Remove from the heat and stir in the cream.
    Refrigerate until needed.

And Finally . . .

It is so wonderful to feel your stomach flat. You have finally got into a whole new way of eating and caring for yourself, and I hope you think it is worth it.

You might still have a way to go. Maybe you have several kilos to lose and it seems daunting. Don't think of it that way. When you fall out of the habit, or you have gone back to your old ways, get back on track by doing the following:

1 Start again - forget what you have done.

2 Remind yourself of your bottom line.

3 Have you gone to the person you told?
   Call him or her - don't wallow, have a cheery chat.

4 Get out and exercise.

5 Congratulate yourself - for each simple thing you do on your midline.

Respect yourself, respect others and respect food. Above all, never fall into the trap of believing the 'hype' about not being able to lose weight after forty or never having a flat stomach after a baby. You will. Remember your bottom line and . . .

Good luck!